Additional Praise for *The Body Hea~ ~~~~*

"*The Body Heals Itself* is a fascinating read. It takes us into the emotions and deep wisdom of our body in surprising ways. This book gives us tools to understand this hidden part of ourselves—one that may have formally been an acquaintance now becomes an intimate friend."

—Dr. Paulette Kouffman Sherman, psychologist and author
of *The Book of Sacred Baths*

"Emily unravels the art of touch and its ties to our deeply held emotions with well-oiled grace. Inspire and be released—one muscle at a time."

—Micah A. Howard MD, CHt, integrative and functional healthcare practitioner,
board certified family physician, master clinical hypnotherapist,
and CEO of Invested Healer, LLC

"Emily is a highly skilled and effective therapist … I highly recommend this book to all athletes and anyone looking to know the body in a more conscious and meaningful way."

—Lara Sturm, USA Powerlifting National Champion
and American record holder

"[Emily Francis] has done her homework in talking with many experts in the field. The materials here are the start of a great new field of study and it makes me want to learn more."

—Craig Marker, PhD, Chair, Mercer University
Clinical Medical Psychology

"Emily Francis allows any residual perceptions of the mind and body in isolation to evaporate. She, literally, merges the concepts of the emotional being and the muscular system that supports, protects, and propels the body. She effectively integrates Eastern and Western medicine, breaking down walls of misunderstanding."

—Sara Raiser, MD, CMT

The
Body
*Heals
Itself*

About the Author

Emily A. Francis is the coauthor of *Witchy Mama: Magickal Traditions, Motherly Insights & Sacred Knowledge* with Melanie Marquis (Llewellyn 2016) and author of *Stretch Therapy: A Comprehensive Guide to Basic and Assisted Stretching* (Blue River Press 2012).

Emily holds a degree in Exercise Science and Wellness with a minor in Nutrition from Jacksonville State University, where she is now pursuing her master's degree in Physical Education with a concentration in Human Performance. She is a graduate of the Atlanta School of Massage in Clinical and Neuromuscular Massage Therapy. She then went on to graduate through all levels of training at the Dr. Vodder School International in Manual Lymphatic Drainage and Combined Decongestive Therapy (MLD/CDT). She is a Certified Pediatric Therapist through Tina Allen and The Liddle Kidz Foundation. She has completed both level 1 & 2 of CranioSacral Therapy through the Upledger Institute.

Emily completed three hundred hours of yoga teacher training through the Universal Yoga Training in the Sivananda Yoga style. She began practicing both yoga and tai chi in the late 1990s and has a gold medal in tai chi forms from the 2001 US Open, a bronze medal in push hands from the same competition, and a silver medal in push hands from the National Tai Chi Legacy tournament that same year. She is a Usui and Karuna Ki Reiki Master level practitioner as well.

You can find Emily at www.emilyafrancisbooks.com.

The
Body
Heals
Itself

❧

How *Deeper Awareness* of Your
Muscles and Their *Emotional*
Connection Can *Help You Heal*

EMILY A. FRANCIS

Llewellyn Publications
Woodbury, Minnesota

FIRST EDITION
Fourth Printing, 2020

Cover design by Ellen Lawson
Interior illustrations by Mary Ann Zapalac
Thank you to Tom Daugherty and Cardinal Publishers for granting permission to include the photos from
    Stretch Therapy

Llewellyn Publications is a registered trademark of Llewellyn Worldwide Ltd.

Library of Congress Cataloging-in-Publication Data
Names: Francis, Emily A., author.
Title: The body heals itself : how deeper awareness of your muscles and their
    emotional connection can help you heal / Emily A. Francis.
Description: First Edition. | Woodbury, Minnesota : Llewellyn Publications,
    2017. | Includes bibliographical references and index.
Identifiers: LCCN 2017035439 (print) | LCCN 2017043158 (ebook) | ISBN
    9780738753515 (ebook) | ISBN 9780738750736 (alk. paper)
Subjects: LCSH: Muscles--Psychological aspects.
Classification: LCC QP321 (ebook) | LCC QP321 .F76 2017 (print) | DDC
    612.7/4--dc23
LC record available at https://lccn.loc.gov/2017035439

Llewellyn Worldwide Ltd. does not participate in, endorse, or have any authority or responsibility concerning private business transactions between our authors and the public.

All mail addressed to the author is forwarded, but the publisher cannot, unless specifically instructed by the author, give out an address or phone number.

Any Internet references contained in this work are current at publication time, but the publisher cannot guarantee that a specific location will continue to be maintained. Please refer to the publisher's website for links to authors' websites and other sources.

Llewellyn Publications
A Division of Llewellyn Worldwide Ltd.
2143 Wooddale Drive
Woodbury, MN 55125-2989
www.llewellyn.com

Printed in the United States of America

Other Books by Emily A. Francis

Witchy Mama

Stretch Therapy: A Comprehensive Guide to Basic and Assisted Stretching
(Blue River Press)

Dedication

This book would not be possible without my teachers: Every professor, instructor, colleague, and client have all been and continue to be my teachers. I am forever grateful.

To my amazing family: You are my everything. You are my heart. I thank you all for your constant love and support.

To Scott: Thank you for being my greatest champion and love.

To God/The Universe/Great Spirit/The Creator of All That Is: My gratitude is ever present.

Acknowledgments

I have so many people to thank for making this book what it is. I thank you all at the Upledger Institute—John Matthew Upledger, Jackie Halderman, Mariann Sisco, Stan Gerome, and Tad Wanveer—for an incredible and life-altering experience.

Additional schools that helped with this project:

The Georgia Massage School

Kripalu Center for Yoga & Health

The Southwest Institute of Healing Arts

Pensacola School of Massage

Everest Schools of Massage Therapy

Individual acknowledgments: Melanie Marquis, Brad Smith, Stephen Watson, Abdi Assadi, MS, Lic, Dr. Paul Epstein, Dr. John Hammett, Dr. Craig Marker, Dr. Alex Alverson, Dr. Sara Raiser, Laura Spucches, William Adcock, L.Ac, David Mitchell, L.Ac, Heather Hale, Laurie Craig, Janie Richardson, Pamela Bellamy, L.Ac, Rick Garbowski, Laura Sturm, Alina Frank, Cheryl Speen, Sherry Leetham, Alyssa Phillips, Laura Allen, Ashli Callaway, Stephanie Colletti, Stanley Keleman, and Shyamala Strack. Thank you Thom Rutledge, Dr. Micah A. Howard, Katie Silcox, Arthur Fretwell, Carola Rodina, Danica Todd, Shaye Hudson MA, LPC, CHt, Liz Kotch, Tom Dill, and Dr. Paulette Kouffman Sherman. Thank you Dattattreya, my yoga teacher, for changing my life in all the best ways. Thank you to Tom Daugherty and Cardinal Publishers for granting permission to include the photos from *Stretch Therapy*. Thank you to my tai chi teachers (all of you) for giving me a deeper understanding of a million things. My heartfelt thanks to each person and school who participated in this survey. If I've left anyone out, my sincere apologies.

Thank you to my literary agent: Paul Levine

Bio Photo: Jessica Allen

Stretch Photos: Kyler Dennis

Thank you to my editors: Angela Wix and Stephanie Finne

Contents

Exercise List

List of Affirmations

Chapter 3

I ask the white light to surround me now.

I am safe, protected, and loved.

I am in a safe, healing space and all actions lead to my greatest good and highest joys.

Peace and healing to all involved.

Chapter 4

I no longer need to carry the weight of the world on my shoulders.

I give what I have when I can with no expectations placed upon myself to give more than this.

I give all I am able without attachment.

I am doing the best I can with what I have where I am and so is everybody else.

I release shames and angers from the past.

I am free to move on without carrying any old knife wounds. The scars may remain, but there is no more pain within them.

I have removed the knife from my back, and I am free to move into the greatest joys of life with no need to ever look back.

I can now express my love freely.

I am love. I give love. I am open to receive love.

I am strong and I am supple.

I move forward in my life with grace and dignity.

I am flexible, willing, and able.

I move freely with ease.

I trust the process.

I am in alignment with Divine guidance.

I am able to move forward with my life without fear of financial worry.

The Universe will provide for me, and I will do my part in my own success.

I take responsibility for my life and my choices with grace and gratitude.

I have love in my heart and joy in my body as I embrace change and fluid motion of forward movement.

I am open and available to heal from the deepest depths of my being *now*.

Chapter 5

I am free to let go of all the times I did not honor my feelings and sat them out.

I embrace a new way of communicating, where I speak my truth freely and kindly so that things do not fester within my being.

I am free to move into a higher space of consciousness.

Angers and frustrations no longer have a place to be planted within me.

I release the frustrations and walk away with ease and peace.

Chapter 6

I am *able*.

I am moving in the direction of my goals.

I am able to run free and move my body in alignment with my heart and mind.

I am an open conduit for love and forward motion in my life.

I am strong, and I am powerful.

I trust my path.

Chapter 7

I am *safe now*.

I am secure.

I affirm that my body is healthy, and I am in rhythm with my body.

I go with the flow and not against it.

I trust my gut to lead me to the highest outcome possible.

I am strong in my body and in my thoughts.

I trust. I am in the flow. I believe in *me*.

Chapter 8

I am *strong*.

I am supple, and I am able to defend my life, my positions, and my beliefs.

I allow negativity to roll off me.

I embrace the really great offerings of life.

I embrace my body, my heart, and my life.

I am open to receiving life's many bountiful blessings.

I am worthy to receive.

I stand with my arms open, my chest open, and my heart open to receive blessings and goodness. I am free to choose happiness.

I allow myself to feel good and experience joy.

I am balanced and stable.

I am strong, and I only allow things to enter my field that are for my highest good and greatest joy.

I resist negativity in my field now.

I grab hold of the good things in my life.

Chapter 9

I am *love*.

I am an all-encompassing being of pure love and joy.

I radiate kindness and compassion for myself and others.

I am open to receiving and giving love without attachment.

I choose love as my primary emotion.

Chapter 10

I *express*.

I allow myself to be honest and forthcoming with information.

I do not hold back my own feelings or emotions.

I do not speak harshly, but I do speak truthfully.

I acknowledge that the muscles of facial expression reveal my feelings.

I allow myself to feel freedom throughout my entire being.

I no longer hang on to things and chew on the bone that no longer serves me.

Chapter 11

I *synthesize.*

I am willful in the most glorious way.

I see the good in life.

I chew and swallow with accuracy any situation life throws at me.

I commit to seeing the whole picture.

I am *flexible.*

I can see life clearly.

I do not bury my head in the sand.

I see the world around me in all its glories and its messes.

I *trust.*

I know that things go on behind me. I trust my own intuition and the world around me.

I am strong, capable, and aware.

I trust that my inner guides always have my back.

Chapter 12

In this moment, every cell in my body corrects itself. Every strand of DNA is recomposed, straightened, and healed.

Any parts of me that have been out of balance restore themselves *now.*

I am healed at the deepest cellular level.

I agree to move forward while trusting my body, my heart, and my mind.

I am now able to live the life I have always imagined I could.

I ask that this be so … And So It Is.

The Missing Piece of the Puzzle: Holistic Healing and the Emotional Muscle Body

Recently I went to a Korean sauna and received an acupressure massage from a man who was quite thorough, did not speak English, and landed on some points on my body that made me realize a basic concept. I had the same questions that I think most people do when they lie on a table in their most vulnerable position, the questions being: What is going through your head right now? What are you feeling? Why does that spot make me want to throw up? Why do you keep returning to that spot? What is that spot? I want to know everything you are thinking while you are treating me! What did you find? Am I healthy?

For me, body work is not relaxing. Parts of it can be and pleasure is generally woven into the treatment; however, much of the time is spent deep breathing, trying not to hold on to whatever is trying to be let out, and constantly wondering what the body worker might know about you by having their hands on you.

The body itself is a master communicator. Since time immemorial, people have attempted to translate its messages, describing and documenting the body's energetic makeup in hopes of discovering the secrets to great health and longevity. In traditional Chinese medicine, the organs all have corresponding emotions, times of day where they are at their strongest and weakest, and even food flavor profiles that pair to the organ. In Ayurvedic medicine (*Ayurveda* is a Sanskrit word meaning "the complete knowledge for long life"), we are divided into three doshas, or body types, that correlate with different foods, different emotions, and different energies. In neuromuscular massage therapy, there's a concept called trigger points, which is a philosophy that aims to explain the phenomenon of *referring pain*, a term used to describe a feeling of pain in one area of the body when pressure is placed on another area of the body. In reflexology, we have the entire body all mapped out on our feet! If the kidney point on the foot hurts, for instance, it could be a sign of kidney duress. There are literally tons of materials and resources available to help us understand the body's energy patterns, chakras, nerve centers, and more. There is one avenue, however—and a major one—that has yet to be explored: the muscles.

Applied kinesiology, or muscle testing, uses the muscles to tap into the subconscious mind. The muscles test stronger or weaker depending on the questions being asked. You can perform muscle testing to find out a host of things—emotional issues, physical pains, sensitivities, etc. For example, my child was on a very strict diet in accordance with results from testing her stool sample. She is not allergic to anything, but we were given a long list of foods that create sensitivities for her. We sought out a naturopath (holistic doctor) to perform something called Nambudripad's allergy elimination technique (NAET). He did a series of muscle tests to see what foods she might be sensitive to, and his results from testing her muscles gave us exactly the same information as our very expensive traditional medical test. (As a side note, this treatment worked for us and we no longer have to keep to that strict diet.)

I share this to say to those who have never realized that the muscles are a part of the body's communicating system, think about the muscle-testing procedures and you may realize that there are many ways to approach our bodies for information and for healing. The muscles are a great resource into the body's deep intelligence. Why then wouldn't we come to see that the muscles themselves hold emotional information as well?

The muscles hold a vast amount of information about our bodies and our emotional state of being. Although the body is a master communicator, we are not master listeners. This book will open your ears as well as your eyes to many avenues of emotional and physical health and healing available to you, and you'll learn how to truly listen to your own emotional muscle body. In discovering how to "hear" and understand what your muscles are telling you, you'll be armed with new knowledge and insight to help keep yourself in the highest state of health and emotional wellness possible.

How This Book Came About

I began formulating the ideas behind this book from early on in massage school when my teacher told us that the psoas and the longus colli were the two most "emotional muscles" in the body. This means that by manually treating these muscles an emotional response was more likely to occur. I became instantly fascinated with what that meant and curious to know more. When I asked my teacher what else in the body is emotional or how do they even know that those two muscles are emotional, he had no answer. It seems that this information has simply been passed down through the generations of body workers as something we should know without worrying about any particular detail or dynamics of the concept.

I was determined to find out as much as I could about this. As I began to work on bodies, this subject matter became all the more necessary to my work. I realized that having an understanding of the body map with regard to treating the muscles and how they pair with emotions is incredibly helpful. Having this knowledge allows me to be able to treat the body with a deeper respect. I began to ask various people about this subject and, as it turned out, many people in the healing field all had little bits and pieces to add to the puzzle.

Ultimately, when it comes to the true backbone of this book however, it is what I found myself, through countless clients' bodies revealing this information to me. I developed an understanding of how to read the body. I began to almost speak to the muscles themselves, or at the very least I learned how to listen to the muscles as they revealed their secret language to me.

As I came forward with what I was formulating, I was given confirmation time and time again by others in this field. For example, later in this book when we discuss Emotional Freedom Technique (EFT), we will find that they already knew that betrayal is held behind the shoulder blades. I knew this same information, but I had never read it anywhere. The body had taught me independently. To have confirmations such as these was invigorating, and they helped me to be able to come forward with confidence that what I offer in this book is valid.

During the process of writing this book, I turned to many teachers and highly respected people in the field. I wanted to reach out to those who would directly disagree with the concepts in this book as well as the ones who have spent their entire career in alignment with this work. I wanted to do this work true justice, and that means seeing it from all sides.

One such counter perspective came from a very well-respected massage educator and author who said, "People look for deeper meaning when there is not any. I too have seen many transformations and healing take place, and I cannot attribute them to anything other than the person was ready for change and that getting them out of chronic pain may have been the catalyst for that." Nothing is an exact science and the body is fully capable of having several options for answers in the areas of distress patterns as well as release methods. These are things we will learn more about in the pages to come.

The Body Heals Itself: Muscle and Emotional Release

I cannot repeat this enough: *the body heals itself.* Your ability to heal is so much greater than anyone has led you to believe. It's just really difficult to do it alone. Everyone needs someone to help them along the path to a new way of being. What you might be looking for is a psychotherapist, a counselor, a chiropractor, a physical therapist, a massage therapist, a Reiki master, or an acupuncturist who knows what it is you are looking for. I hope that by the end of this book you will have a clearer idea of the kinds of people you need to seek out for what your body and your mind need at this time.

The muscles store emotional memory. They do not create, produce, or move the emotions. It is through the muscle/mind connection that the emotions that are stored within the muscle fibers and fascia (the thin, fibrous tissue that surrounds the muscles) are able to be moved and released. The muscles do not have their own mind; the mind is the mind. The muscles simply store what the body has endured throughout its life—this is both great memories as well as traumatic memories.

In Western society, we view the muscles as our physical driving force, our source of strength—and not much else beyond that. The study of the muscles focuses on chemical makeup, origin, insertion, and functions. We even know the fiber directions of every muscle in the body. But do we have any idea that the muscles themselves hold a highly emotional part of our being? Do we know that our muscles can tell us very early on what parts of our emotional body needs to be addressed and treated? When we learn to listen to our muscles, we can discover emotional and physical problems sooner, before it's too late to do anything about them. When we understand the emotional muscle body as a whole, we're empowered to change the patterns of our lives for the better.

Understanding your body's muscular system on an emotional level is not about weight lifting and learning how to build strength and muscle mass, nor is it essential to memorize the many chemical compounds and trigger points that exist within those muscles. What's needed is a road map to the muscles, exploring not just their physical aspects but their emotional and spiritual components as well. This book will take you on an emotional and energetic journey within your own body. It's time to unlock the mysteries of what the muscles know and hold for you. It's time to use this knowledge to improve your health, your mood, and your life.

I worked with a woman on and off for several years. One day when she came in for a massage session, she was in a great mood. We chatted for just a little bit, and then I proceeded to work on her muscles. I started her on her back, facing up. I had already finished the whole front side of her body. There was nothing too noticeable anywhere and certainly no emotions flaring up. I turned her over and worked on her legs first and then got to the gluteus, or the buttocks area. All of a sudden, her muscles became so tight that it was very painful and difficult for me to continue to work on her. And she didn't want me to, either! In fact, she was getting aggravated, hoping I would just skip past the tense area. She got angry with me. I had to be going too deep. What was the deal? I didn't let up. I knew what was coming. This was not just something physical at all. It was emotional.

I know that the buttocks holds aggravation and suppression. You know those times when something makes you angry but you know it's just not worth talking about, so you sit on it… You literally do sit on it, and the emotions enter into the glutes. It's no wonder she was experiencing aggravation as I treated this area. The emotions that it stored were coming to surface. Without any coaxing, and although she was feeling very aggravated with the massage, she lifted her head up, turned to me, and said: "Did I tell you that my ex-husband just died? Did I tell you about his new wife and all the trouble she's caused?" Now, why would this all of a sudden come up in conversation—in the conversation that we weren't having? One minute, we were talking about "Why does this hurt so much here?" and the next minute she blurts out, "Did I tell you that my ex-husband just died?" I was massaging her buttocks, exactly where all of her frustration and aggravation were sitting! Of course she would bring this up right then! Now we were getting to it so she could let it go. The physical pain that was in that area began to subside as she talked.

Getting that area treated physically and at the same time discussing the emotional component made the pent-up pain leave. It did not have to fester into something that would become worse. It was gone. Acknowledging and understanding the emotional pain that was felt through the physical pain was truly liberating for this woman, and this is just one little story in a long line of real-life examples. This is one very simple story because the emotions were fresh. It was an easy release. But what happens when the muscles have been holding on to serious pain, anger, shame, and sorrow for years on end?

Certain muscles guard certain emotions, but it's not always as straightforward as it might sound. When you press on one muscle and they feel pain in another part, that is known as referral pain from a trigger point. There is an emotional component to that as well. It is the part I call the Apothecary Method. When you are working on an area that doesn't just hold trigger points and referral pains but something deeper and more emotional, the client will unknowingly stuff it into another part of their body, hoping you will miss it. It is your job to keep opening the drawers of the body to find out where that little rascal slipped off to in order to hide itself.

There are trigger points and referral pain charts everywhere, but the emotional part is not on any referral pattern chart. This is something entirely different. People don't want to face old pains. It is not comfortable. They don't even consciously realize that they still hold that old pain. They don't acknowledge that they never actually faced whatever the trauma or issue was, which leads to the concept that by not facing it, it was never released. So it sits and waits to be found or prefers never to be found. We must go after it and wage a small yet more sensitive war on the little rascal so you can escort it kindly out of the body forever.

Anytime that we get our hearts broken or we witness a terrible loss, we tuck away those emotions somewhere in our minds to postpone the pain until a later date. We deal with what we can, and we hide the rest. It's simply human nature. But I believe that when that place in your mind gets overcrowded, it calls on its resources to hang on to it too—the muscles, the fascia, the organs, and further out into the energy fields. It has to go somewhere!

What happens to the things that you've stuffed into your little "soul drawers" along the way? Where are they now? When emotional pains aren't processed and dealt with completely, they lie dormant in the body until there is just no room for them in the sock drawers of your soul and they must come out. Unfortunately, these sleeping monsters generally come forward through physical pain or illness. This is the emotional root of dis-ease. This is not to say that dis-ease doesn't primarily have physical, lifestyle, and genetic causes, because it clearly does, but it does sometimes have an emotional component as well that can warn us in advance to the onset of illness so that we can pursue treatment before it gets worse. When we don't listen, or when we don't even know what to listen for, we run the risk of getting sick. Illness is the final way that our body lets us know that we are out of sync. Before it gets to the point where the emotional pain manifests itself into something physical, the body sends all kinds of warning signals in an attempt to alert us to the fact that our body and soul are in need of attention.

One of our primary security systems for letting us know when the body is in disorder is the muscular system. By noticing how our muscles feel and behave, we can nip illness and physical discomfort in the bud and liberate ourselves from old emotional tensions and sorrows that have held us back. In understanding the energetic body as a whole and how it relates to the emotional muscle body, you'll gain the key to becoming the greatest authority on your own health, and you'll have the tools you need to overcome any emotional or spiritual obstacles along the way. Knowledge is power, and it's time you had yours in knowing your own body.

It is important to note, however, that not every single thing in your muscles comes down to an emotional pain that has been hiding out. Sometimes it really is just physical, or repetitive habits. Sometimes your shoulders hurt not necessarily because you are dealing with the weight of the world on your shoulders or feeling like no one else can do it like you can ... sometimes it really is that your purse is ridiculously heavy and you don't change arms! While what I am offering here is incredible information, it is not the only suggestion for what might be going on in your muscular body. There are too many times that we can get carried away with our holistic views and miss some very simple things.

Use this knowledge to broaden your perspective, and continue to keep your ears open to every way in which the body speaks.

Wherever in your body you have muscle pains, especially ongoing muscle pains, can reveal the emotional components that are currently in your life or were experienced in the past and left unprocessed. If you have an acute pain in your body, this does not automatically represent some sort of long-held betrayal. It may mean that something new has come up—something that may or may not be attached in any way to something old. Or it could be as simple as you moved in a weird way and the physical muscle seized up. You must go through the full list of possibilities—the physical as well as the emotional.

Are you stretching, taking care of your body, honoring your thoughts, eliminating the negative patterns in your life? Are you wearing good shoes? Do you carry stress? Do you discuss things that bother you? Do you stuff them down deep and these things are now being triggered? These questions should be part of your body scan. The mind is still the processing organism in the body, and I do not believe you can accurately release the muscles of emotions without the mind being at the wheel. You can release muscle tissue of chronic tightness, of spasms, of anything physical—yes, of course! But I am going deeper and into the area that *does* require the mind to be part of the discussion and of the movement—into lasting healing that helps not only the body but also the mind, heart, and soul. Other therapists who work with body energy and release patterns already know this. This is not a new concept. It's just that so far, only small articles and little bits and pieces have been shared throughout the years. No one has managed to put it all together comprehensively in book form.

How to Use This Book

What this book ultimately is encouraging you to do is look beyond what you know and allow your body to heal and to access not only the traumas for release but the good and the joys to increase health and vitality within your being. As we go along, we will learn the various muscle groups and what emotion is likely stored in this particular area. The mind must be a fully active part of healing, working together with the rest of the body, including the muscles themselves, to completely transform. Once we do so, we're empowered to move forward into our healthiest form of living.

Allow the knowledge and tools you will acquire throughout this book to help bring you into the highest joys of your life no matter what your age and no matter what health you are in currently. There are so many available ways to heal, and this happens to be one of them. The mind/muscle connection can be an important aspect of healing, and no longer will I allow this part to be overlooked.

In the muscle chapters, I will offer stretches, affirmations, and visualizations to help connect yourself to the muscles that can assist with self-release. Throughout this book, I will offer affirmations, visualizations, meditations, stones, and essential oils that pair with the muscle or emotion that help with healing the emotions.

Prayer: When we pray, we talk a lot and focus on things we need and are asking for. Hopefully in prayer we are also giving thanks.

Centering: When we center ourselves, it is a way to calm our minds so that answers may be received in response to our prayers and questions.

Meditation: Meditation is a space offered to help you get into a place within your mind that allows for your mind, body, and spirit to come together for your highest space to blend into one consciousness. Going deeper beyond simply centering our minds and bodies can lead us to meditation. Meditation to me is the art of doing nothing. You are no longer engaged in your thoughts. You are not asking for anything. You can enter a space where time slows down. It lends itself to a freedom from deep within your being to calm, quiet, and accept love energy from outside yourself as well as deep within your own being.

The word *meditation* throws a lot of people off due to the complexity that it can be. The idea behind meditation is to get to a still point in your mind where you are virtually doing nothing. It is the place that you can get to that transcends all thoughts, mind chatter, and outside distractions and brings you to a place of supreme bliss. For the purpose of this book, in any meditation or centering practice, it is a stepping back and becoming only an observer of your thoughts without an attachment. You no longer engage in the chatter simply by being still in your body and calming your mind and detaching from any distractions in the path.

Affirmations: When it comes to affirmations, these are statements to be repeated to yourself to help to solidify the new attitude for various areas to heal itself. Repeating positive statements becomes affirmative in nature. This is an important component in your journey. Affirmations are short enough that you can remember the statement easily so you are able to repeat it with ease throughout your day. As I list various affirmation options, whichever statement resonates best with you is the one to choose.

Visualizations: A visualization is like a meditation in motion. I will lead you through imagery to help you picture in your mind your body engaging in release and healing. As you go through them, truly try to visualize yourself going through each suggestion to get to a more comfortable place within your body.

Stones: Crystals and gemstones come naturally with healing properties. An example of this would be rose quartz, which is known for the unconditional love energy that the stone carries. In this text, I will offer various stones that can be the most beneficial to the area we are discussing. In the back of the book in appendix A, I will discuss how to clean your stones and which stones are best for grounding, healing, releasing, renewal, etc. In the chapters on the muscles as well as the chakras, I will include stones to pair with the area.

Essential Oils: When we discuss essential oils, the safest method of use is to drop the oil in a diffuser that contains water. This way the oils are misting into the air and can be enjoyed by everyone. When applying to the skin, it is always a better idea to mix the oil with a carrier oil such as coconut oil, jojoba oil, or grapeseed oil. Add only a small number of drops as a 3:1 ratio of carrier oil to essential oil. If you are doing a tablespoon of carrier oil, maybe add three drops of essential oil. Some oils such as lavender, ylang ylang, and jasmine (the calmer, softer oils) can be applied directly in small amounts to the skin. Oils such as peppermint, eucalyptus, and spearmint (the more revitalizing scents) should not be applied on the skin without dilution.

In appendix A, I offer recipes for detox baths, as well as more information on crystals and how to use them and take care of them. Breathing practices (pranayama) will be in that section as well.

In appendix B, I have several different people write deeper explanations of the various modalities that I list in this text. I have information on Ayurveda, Chinese medicine, tapping technique, Bach flower remedies, toe reading, a lesson in forgiveness, and more. I offer these to provide deeper insight into these subjects that can help us on our journey. As I've moved along in compiling the information for this book, I have interviewed so many incredibly generous people. All of the people who offer their expertise give way to a deeper awareness of the body and the avenues in which to help the body heal itself. You will be able to hear from some of the greatest experts in this field, and I have been honored that they would grant me their time and their information with such love and willingness to teach us all.

I met Stephen Watson, world champion martial artist, in Sedona at a tai chi workshop many years ago. He was one of the teachers there. This is the first time I had ever met someone who spends more time of the night in meditation than in sleep. He teaches meditation classes all over the world. (Please see appendix B for his well-worn and life-tested instructions that are designed to be simple yet comprehensive.) This is one example of what is offered in the appendix section of this book.

I want to take you on a quest to learn more about body healing and body awareness. I believe that *the body heals itself*, and we are never the healers. When we help someone, whether it's through massage or physical therapy or through energy work or emotional release, we are not the ones doing the healing. We are simply the open vessel through which sacred healing energy may flow. A person must be open and willing to heal, and most of the time this is achieved through understanding what needs to heal and from where the problem is issuing.

We know a lot of emotional places in the mind, we know a lot of emotional places in our hearts... but it's time we learn of those emotional places that reside in the rest of the body, within the muscles. The body is splendid, and it is a mystery we must learn to discover.

Use this information in good health, friends. Use this as an addition to your practice and your understanding of your own body and the bodies of others. Use this with an open mind and, above all, an open heart. May we all learn that our body tells our story. Our bodies do speak our minds, our hearts, our traumas, our celebrations, and our perceptions of the world. Let our minds and our bodies finally unite in a strong and healthy way that guides us into a deeper level of healing.

I am truly honored to share this journey with you.
In full body wellness and love, I offer this work.
—Emily A. Francis

Part I

The Connection between Emotions and Our Muscles

Chapter 1

Muscles, Memory,
Emotions, and the Link

This chapter offers a brief breakdown of the muscular system. It's important to have our muscle basics down so that we can understand the possibility of the muscles being able to store emotions and the role they play in emotional healing throughout the entire body.

When you look at a dandelion, what do you see? Some look at the golden dandelion and see amazing healing properties for body detoxification. Dandelion greens are packed with nutrients such as calcium and iron. The roots, the leaves, and the stems of a dandelion are all useful to us and have been used in medicine and food for as long as we can trace back. From a spiritual perspective, it is believed that the yellow petals represent the sun, while the white puff dandelion represents the moon. When you blow out the white puffs, it is seen as the stars. To others, they see these flowers as a nuisance and a weed. It's all about perspective.

The way that each person views the body is much the same as the way someone could view a dandelion. Some see the body separate from the brain and only give focus to the brain or the mind. Some see the body from a looks perspective and not much deeper than this. Some people view the muscles as your source of strength. Many don't think beyond what the muscles look like unless they are taught how to work with the muscles. When I was in school, the way that my teachers would scan someone's body in two seconds flat was baffling to me. Now, as a bodyworker, I do it all the time. I scan everyone that I come in contact with. The way that I look at the whole body is completely different than it ever was before.

Someone who only works with one area of practice tends to keep the perspective to that one item. If someone treats you through cognitive therapy, that is how they will scan your whole body. How you respond verbally, as well as your physical movements, correlate to what they know about your emotional space from a mind perspective. A personal trainer will watch how you move with a completely different vision. They will watch how you move to formulate the plan of how to train your muscles to look their best. Again, it is all about the perspective from which you are seeing the opportunities to heal. Our goal here is to view the body from an emotional perspective through the eyes of physical awareness. Your muscles store emotions, and where you carry pain and tension can provide great details of your physical, emotional, and mental health.

The Muscular System

Let's begin with a simple muscle breakdown. There are more than six hundred muscles in the human body. The primary purpose of the muscles is movement of the body. There are three types of muscle:

1. Cardiac muscles: Cardiac muscles are the involuntary muscles that make up the heart. These muscles operate without our conscious control.

2. Smooth muscles: These are the muscles found in organ systems, such as the digestive and respiratory systems. The smooth muscles are also involuntary muscles that operate without your conscious control to keep you alive.

3. Skeletal muscles: Skeletal muscles are what we usually think of when we refer to muscles—biceps, calves, abs, and so on. These are voluntary muscles because we have to make a conscious decision to make them move. This is done through the nervous system. The nervous system receives and responds to move the muscle through the stimulation of the nerves themselves.

Each muscle has a specific nerve or nerve bundle that runs through it. The nerves send signals throughout the body via the central nervous system (CNS). The CNS is the body's messaging system. When we experience anything happy, sad, painful, etc., we feel it physically through our central nervous system. The CNS consists of the brain and spinal cord, and this is where the link between muscle, nerve, and emotions comes to life. My studies go further than simply saying that through nerves and body signals one is able to experience emotions through palpations of the muscles. Going one step further, through working with countless bodies and also discussing this subject with several people in this or related fields, my hypothesis is that each muscle group within the body carries associations with specific emotional patterns. Each particular group of muscles tends to have a certain emotion that is associated with that particular area of the body.

The nervous system is the window to the muscles. Each movement of the muscle goes hand in hand with the nervous system. If there is a disconnect between the two, it can result in an inability to move that muscle or area. This is what we refer to as paralysis. Let that sink in. These muscles move after a conscious thought to make them move. That sentence alone should easily tie the brain to the muscles for movement and tie the mind to the muscles for the thought. They all work hand in hand. Nothing within the body operates by itself.

The supportive structures for the muscles are tendons, ligaments, and fascia. Tendons connect muscle to the bone. Fascia is a band of connective tissue that attaches, stabilizes, and separates muscles as well as the body organs. Ligaments, like fascia, are comprised of connective tissue and connect bone to other bones. Fascia requires a bit deeper understanding. As my teacher described, fascia is like the body's panty hose. Fascia is everywhere in the body with different densities of the matrix.

Life Force Energy

Chi/Qi in China, in Japan it is pronounced *KI*, and in India it is known as *prana*, all translate into the same definition: life force energy. In the United States, we have no such word or term for this. In the Eastern traditions, the body and the mind never did separate as a belief, so they are thousands of years ahead in full body awareness. In the West, we separated the body from the mind long ago, which results in a lack of understanding and a lack of application to keep the body grounded and united. We deal in sick care mostly here in the West. They deal with well care mostly as well as preventative care in the East.

The life force energy is believed to be breathed into you the moment you were born. That same life force energy was breathed into every single living cell, animal, or person.

This is the foundation of life. When you think of your body, imagine it more like moving water. The arms and legs have water hoses running through each limb of the body. Any blockage or bend in a hose causes the water to get blocked and stop running. That is the same idea behind the chi. Meridian channels that run through the body carry the chi. This is much like the bloodstream carries blood to the different parts of your body. When we have stagnant chi, our energy body gets blocked and backed up. It is believed that in the physical sense, the chi runs through the fascia of the body.

When I began working on this book, I spoke with several professionals. I met with resistance when it came to understanding energetic and emotional differences between muscles and fascia. One person said that looking at the muscle without thinking of the fascia was like taking the water out of the river. In Chinese medicine, there are meridian channels that run throughout the body. The way that it was explained to me, with reference to fascia and the meridians themselves, was that the chi (life force energy) is conducted along the matrix of the fascia. With meridian channels, the energy is either feminine (yin) or masculine (yang). The yin and yang must remain balanced with each other to maintain good health. The energy flows through the meridian channels throughout the body. (See appendix B for further information on Chinese medicine and meridian channels.)

I had an interview with a very gifted author, speaker, and practitioner of Chinese medicine/acupuncture, Abdi Asadi MS, Lic. Ac, about this very subject. He said, "The body has intelligence. In our culture, the body is considered low level. We are brain dominant. People don't understand that the body holds so much information. We view the body to be submissive to the brain. But the body stores everything. It's like a CD-ROM downloaded and stored in the fascia. That is where the chi runs through. We are very geared toward the brain, but the body has intelligence."

When it comes to healing the body, Asadi has found that because we are so brain dominant, we commit ourselves to what we perceive as truths that don't actually resonate with the body.

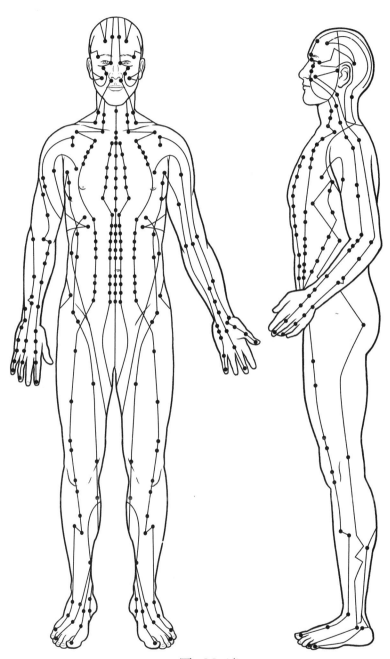

The Meridians

"People don't want the truth, but the body doesn't lie," he says. "People become so committed to the lie and the masks that they hide behind that they will let their body die. That disconnect is really deep." There is always an emotional component when it comes to physical illness, whether this is cancer, cardiovascular events, and circulation issues. Even dying of a broken heart is entirely possible. Emotions are just as important to any illness and must not be overlooked. Learning new positive attitudes and clearing old painful emotions can lead to miraculous healing when paired with the physical treatments necessary for healing.

There really is no way to treat the muscles without including the fascia. The fascia surrounds the muscle everywhere in the body. However, as its own emotional component and energy being, the muscles themselves are not the same thing as the fascia. They are not made up of the same things. Blood runs through muscle. Blood does not run through fascia.

"The blood carries the emotions and relates to memory," my fellow massage therapist and acupuncturist David Mitchell has stated. Therefore, in this respect the memories carried through the blood and plasma are delivered through the muscles and not through the fascia.

I view fascia as a structure and muscle as a function. You cannot have one without the other, but they are not the same. Emotions and energy do not carry the same way within their structures, either. In my belief, the fascia has the energy running along it, but energy does not burrow down into it the way it can with the muscles. Fascia is like the walls, floor, and ceiling of a room. In the muscles, I believe that energy and emotions bury themselves into the belly of the actual muscle and are a direct connect to the mind. In my vision of the bedroom, the muscles are the bed in the middle of the room. The fascia are the walls, floor, and ceiling that hold up the place.

I met with resistance when introducing muscles into the emotional mix. Due to the literature of Chinese medicine and the five thousand years of study behind it, emotions play a powerful role with the meridians. The meridian channels move directly alongside the fascia that encases muscle and covers the entire body. Fascia and muscle are so connected that it was difficult at first for many to acknowledge that the emotional component is slightly different between the two. I was told that it would be a good idea to expand my understanding of all of this and travel to the Upledger Institute, where CranioSacral Therapy (CST) was founded. There I could learn about structure, function, and the nervous system all in one.

CranioSacral Therapy

At the Upledger Institute, I learned about CranioSacral Therapy. This incredible work addresses the brain, spinal cord, and cerebral spinal fluid. This work is super light with minimal movement but with maximum intention behind it. Knowledge of the brain and spinal cord is necessary for this work. Learning to tune into the body's craniosacral rhythm and then working along with that rhythm in order to help clear space and allow the body to heal itself is the foundation of this work.

I have long since been in awe of the CST work, but only from afar. What I got from my visit to the Upledger Institute was so much more than I ever could have imagined. I met with John Matthew Upledger, the son of the late doctor who had discovered this work, and learned all about his dad and how he came into CST. The doctor had several years of clinical research from the medical center at a major university that led him to discover and support this work. As a jazz musician as well as an osteopath, he had an incredible talent to tune into the body and listen to its unique rhythm.

CST is highly clinical, scientific, and energetic work that requires intense knowledge as well as a true passion for the recipient to heal. As the doctor would say, "We need to listen to a person's body in a way that has never been heard before. Love must be in your hands."

To hear the body's sacred rhythm was astounding to me. While it looks like energy work, and in part it is, it goes so far beyond with intention, knowledge, and listening. The work is intense and the results are wide ranging.

Speaking with their instructors on the subject of fascia versus muscle helped me to define or undefine various ways of discussing the body and how it applies to the muscles storing emotions. I left with a clearer picture and a deeper understanding into fascia, structure, function, and healing.

In their summary with regard to emotion, they said, "Emotion is accessed through the tissue anywhere, and it is up to our inner wisdom to decide what's going to happen." They also said that the doctor never separated fascia and muscle and only referred to it as "tissue memory" because you cannot have one without the other. I find it best to leave it at that. I continue to define the emotions stored based by the category of the muscles themselves, with a deeper understanding that it may very well line up respectively with the meridian channels that also run through the muscles.

Muscle Memory

I want to explain the phenomenon of muscle memory and how it applies to emotions and our muscle body. I spoke with Dr. John Hammett, who is a Doctor of Exercise Physiology and currently the Dean of the College of Education at Jacksonville State University. He said:

> There is something within the neurological pathways that is modified to certain recurring activities by the body. There is a neurological adaptation to repeated activity. Once you have a skill, you will always have that skill. Unless you had an injury, then there could be damage to the neurological pathway and muscle memory might become impaired. The location in which this occurs is in the cerebellum. This is the core of muscle memory. If it is a sport, you must repeat the movement in the correct way to develop the most accurate muscle memory related to a movement. For example, in baseball when they hit the bat to the ball—if they've hit it well—they know what it feels like to knock it out of the park and hit the home run. They know that feeling. It is deeply ingrained into their neurological pathways. You know it when you hit it.
>
> When referring to a trauma, that too becomes locked into the muscle's memory. If you experience anything like it again, you will experience a body reaction to the stimulus. You know to flinch or tighten your body. It doesn't take repetitive times to lock into muscle memory. The motor control and muscle memory comes from the cerebellum. Thought processes are in other parts of the brain.

Research has shown that the amygdala, a small almond-shaped structure deep inside the brain, and the hippocampus, a tiny structure located on both sides of the brain that resembles a sea horse in shape and is part of the limbic system, seem to be the main areas involved with emotions. The amygdala is located in the front portion of the temporal lobes of the brain. There are two amygdala, one on each lobe. A primary function of the amygdala is to connect scent to emotion. The hippocampus is responsible for long- and short-term memory and spatial awareness.

While understanding scientifically that the muscles connect to the brain and neurological pathways that have a direct effect with emotions, we somehow have missed the very basic information that our muscles/tissues/fascia/fluids/plasma are all connected to the whole. If an emotion pairs up with the nervous system, the whole body feels it.

Looking Into Emotion

Now that we have a little more information about the muscles and what they do, we can look at the mind and the cognitive function and how it includes the muscles. I reached out to a former student of mine who is a doctoral candidate in clinical psychology with a focus in neuropsychology. His response to where the muscles might fit in with relation to the mind was very interesting:

> I see the mind and brain as one—that "consciousness" as we know is a by-product of neural activity, not an independent phenomenon. This is relevant to your questions because I don't separate the idea of the "mind" and "body" (the brain being part of the body). Many in my field (myself included) see emotions as being composed of three distinct but related components—thoughts, behaviors, and feelings. Whether or not all of these components are required for "emotion" is debatable, and outside my expertise. In the context of muscles, my first thought is that muscle activity is an external expression of behavior. Since behavior is a component of emotion, it stands that muscles definitely can have a role in emotion. This is supported by experiments where facial muscle activity is manipulated while people read comics (by stimulating muscles necessary for smiling/frowning or by having someone hold a pen between their teeth or lips to mimic a smile or frown, respectively). The findings of studies like this generally show that stimulating or using muscles for smiling leads to people finding the comics to be funnier.
>
> The effect has been found in the opposite direction, where people are injected with Botox (weakening the expression of a smile, for example) and those people report a lesser degree of positive emotion compared to controls. Thus, there is good support for the idea that the state of our bodies influences our experience of emotion.

However, this can't be the only explanation for emotion, since emotions can exist independent from muscle activity/body sensation. People with congenital disorders that leave facial muscles partially paralyzed can still experience happiness.

As for how emotion is processed in the brain, there are many structures and pathways that are important. Most research on emotion shows that there are no areas of the brain that are specific to a certain emotion—that is, any one emotion is associated with activity in many brain regions, and those regions will tend to show activity related to emotion and other functions, such as behaviors (consistent with the definition of emotion as including feelings and behaviors, maybe). From what I can tell, approximately the same systems are active for positive and negative emotion, with the frontal lobes helping to modulate the intensity of emotion by regulating the magnitude of activity in other areas, for example, the amygdala. There is a lot of research to suggest that activity in the left and right frontal lobes is related to separate categories of behavior, which can be associated with emotions—left frontal activity related to approach behaviors (excitement, happiness, but also anger), and right frontal activity related to withdrawal behavior (fear, sadness). In my view, emotions aren't "stored" as much as they are "experienced in response to internal or external stimuli."

The idea that experiences are processed and stored makes sense. Basically, there are a couple things happening: an experience (external stimulus) is associated with a certain pattern of neural activation, in certain circuits. That activity might be associated with positive emotion. Repeated exposure to that stimulus repeatedly activates the same regions and circuits, which over time are strengthened and sometimes expanded. For example, the stronger and better-rehearsed a certain memory is, the greater the extent of brain regions become active when recalling that memory. So memories, like emotions, are not "stored" in one place but are associated with more broad activation. These mechanisms of association explain why memories are stronger when you use more senses to store them. This is also partially why traumatic experiences have such a strong impact.

In summary, pain as well as pleasure is stored not just in the mind but also within the body's tissues. I believe that therapies that work with the mind can help you release the trauma and stored pain as well, and through the muscle/mind connection and releasing through the body you can achieve the same. It is through my own experience that having the body release along with the thoughts is a faster way to get down to it and heal from down deep. With tissue release, information is released as well. The truth is, whether it is done through cognitive skills and therapies or through emotional release and body work, for each person it comes down to whichever method is able to receive the information within to reach the pain and let go of it.

When we go through any sort of shame, fear, guilt, betrayal, or any trauma, it is stored in our minds, in our brains, and in our bodies. Our mind and our brain are not the same thing, and many times they are used interchangeably and they need not be. The mind is where the thoughts live. This is where therapy can help develop the coping skills to help change the mind grooves of beliefs. The brain is an organ. It is made up of chemicals and it is responsible for keeping the body working. When we experience trauma, it goes into our mind and our emotions then trigger the brain, which then releases chemicals. The trauma also goes into the body. The pain has to go somewhere and into the muscles it burrows. Into the energy centers it hides. Into the aura it can show itself. Into every part of our being it becomes. From the emotional standpoint, this is the beginning of physical illness and can manifest into dis-ease if not treated and released from the deepest level of your being.

The Reality of the Body

I sat down for a talk with the world-renowned author, lecturer, and director of Berkeley's Center for Energetic Studies, Stanley Keleman. Among his many books are *Emotional Anatomy* as well *Your Body Speaks Its Mind*. These books were brought to my attention at the beginning of this journey; however, I do not like to read other people's work during my own process of writing. I do not want to sound like other people or be influenced by other people and their work. At the end of my writing process, one of the books again was brought to my attention by someone else. In that moment, I knew it was time to reach out and ask for a sit down, and he was kind enough to give me that honor.

I wanted to know what his idea was behind *Emotional Anatomy*. Keleman believes in a "somatic reality" (Somatic = body, so the reality of the body). The second person who mentioned his work to me had studied with Keleman forty years before. He remembers a time when Keleman taught at a psychiatric conference and made reference to something along the lines of "You don't have to tell me what's going on, I can see it in your body." Keleman and I sat down for a brief talk, and he told me:

Every cell pulsates. The body is a coordinated community of pulsating anatomical structures continually expanding and contracting, like the beating of the heart. Each person's body speaks its own and a universal somatic language, which is communicated in the organizing of and expression of anatomical behaviors that include muscular and cortical activity, intention and feeling, as well as conceiving a future. The organism's primary pulsatory dynamic is its most basic organizing force. This organizing force is expressed in the muscular shapes and cortical configurations (thinking and memory) we mobilize to meet life's challenges.

He said he conceived *Emotional Anatomy* as a pioneering work intended to illustrate the relationships of behavior shapes and emotional attitudes. He continued:

Each body tells of its process and how it supports its life structure and tries to be alive. The human organism has inherited programs, directions for growing itself through all the stages of living, including ways of responding to protect itself and maintain survival. We call these responses instinct or reflex acts. When met with life's challenges, the body may enact its inherited program, but this response may not be the best adaptation for forming a satisfying solution.

He mentioned to me the S shape, which would signal to him that a person may be living in a way that suggests resignation or "I give up." He has identified other common body shapes such as startle, investigation, fight or flight, despair or collapse. He said too often people are undereducated about how to use themselves to intervene and modify problematic behaviors, and that sometimes we are operating on a false belief that our bodies always know the best way to maintain a state of health and healing. Overusing meditation or deep relaxation as a way to effect behavior change has limited success because the body does not always know how to make novel behaviors (which are new anatomical configurations) nor how to support them. That is why a person who feels great after body work may feel terrible again three days later. They don't know how to maintain the new state and continue to support healing on their own unless they learn to use themselves differently. I feel the same way with regard to three days after body work you may be faced with the same challenges unless you find someone to help you to release from a deeper place within.

⌘ Clenching and Relaxing Visualization

Flexing and releasing your muscles is the easiest way to get the body to relax. Taking it slightly deeper with the intention to fully engage with your body allows it to release the tension it carries around without you realizing it is weighted down.

Begin by lying down on your back and closing your eyes. Bring your arms out from the body with your palms facing up. Let the legs also come out from the body and let the feet fall out to each side. Breathe slowly and deeply into the body. Notice your belly rise and expand with each breath in, notice the belly button come back down toward the spine with each breath out. Come into the space of your breath and relax into it. Take a breath in and hold your breath. Tense all of the muscles in your legs and lift your feet an inch off the ground.

As you exhale, relax the legs completely. Let them be heavy, limp. Inhale and hold your breath and tighten every muscle in your arms and make a fist with your hands. Lift your hands one inch off the ground. Exhale and relax the arms and open up the hands, wiggle the fingers. Allow your arms to hang off the body like the arms of a rag doll. No tension. Inhale and hold your breath. Lift your chest and stomach up high, arching the back. Tighten every muscle in the stomach and the back.

Exhale and lower the back down gently, unrolling the vertebrae of the spine down deeply into the floor from the top of the neck to the bottom of the spine. Clench your bottom and relax it, tucking your hips under and allowing your low back to get as close to the ground as possible. Inhale and hold your breath. Lift your head one inch off the ground. Tighten the jaws; shut the eyes tight. Exhale and lower the head down and relax the face. For a second after, open your eyes wide, stick your tongue out, and then relax your face completely and close your eyes. Notice in this space that the entire physical body is relaxed. Breathe deeply into this space, locking into your muscle memory the sensation of being completely and utterly relaxed.

Repeat the following:

- I'm relaxing my feet. My feet are relaxing. My feet are relaxed.
- I'm relaxing my knees. My knees are relaxing. My knees are relaxed.
- I'm relaxing my legs. My legs are relaxing. My legs are relaxed.
- I'm relaxing my hips. My hips are relaxing. My hips are relaxed.
- I'm relaxing my abdomen. My abdomen is relaxing. My abdomen is relaxed.
- I'm relaxing my chest and collar bones. My chest is relaxing. My chest is relaxed.
- I'm relaxing my back. My lower back, my middle back, my upper back are relaxed.
- I'm relaxing my arms and hands. My arms and hands are relaxing. My arms and hands are relaxed.
- I'm relaxing the back of my head. I'm relaxing the top of my head. My head is relaxing. My head is relaxed.
- I'm relaxing my face. My forehead is relaxing. My eyes are relaxing. My cheeks are relaxing. My teeth and tongue are relaxing. My chin is relaxing. My ears are relaxing. My entire face is relaxed.
- I'm relaxing my kidneys, my spleen, and my gallbladder. I'm relaxing my stomach, my intestines, my pancreas, and my liver. I'm relaxing my lungs and my heart. Finally, I am relaxing my brain. My entire body is relaxing. My entire body is relaxed.

Chapter 2

The Emotional, Mental, and Energetic Body

The sacred trinity of the body has been in place forever—the body, mind, and spirit. In yoga, it is referred to as the physical self, the conscious self, and the highest self. Each needs to be acknowledged in its own right, as it takes all of these parts to make up the whole being. The notion of the body as a physical entity is familiar to all of us, but the idea of the body as more than something physical isn't yet fully acknowledged.

If you are a psychologist, psychotherapist, or do any similar work, the emotional body has always been part of the understanding, even if the exact terminology hasn't been in place. If you're a spiritual type of person, you may already have an idea about the spirit body. A person who practices tai chi, yoga, or acupuncture may talk about the energy body and how it connects to the physical body through the sacred life force called chi (China), ki (Japan), or prana (India).

This word does not exist in our Western culture, the energy body is not acknowledged. But our energy body is a vital piece of the whole. Different practitioners and spiritual traditions use different terms to describe the body as an energetic, emotional, physical, or spiritual being. Becoming familiar with these different perspectives will help you develop a greater understanding of the body as a whole.

The Physical Body

Our physical body is the densest of all the body ideas in this text. It is made up of flesh, bones, blood, organs, etc. It is what we can see, touch, and move. It is the vessel we spend this entire life in. It is our current storehouse for our soul. Our physical body defines so much of how we view ourselves. It also is a reflection of the self-care that we practice. To be good to the physical body one needs proper exercise, a nourishing diet, good sleep, and low stress. Our body is our temple. To truly connect with your body, you must take a path of full self-acceptance. Too many times we are taught that we have to be perfect, look this way or that, lose weight, or anything else on the long list of criticisms of our physical self. We are so much more than that!

It is recommended that you be fully engaged in your physical life as much as you might be engaged in your spiritual life but in a different way. Going deeply into your own being and learning to become truly happy with who you are and what you represent to the world opens a door to supreme bliss. I don't believe you can achieve this without a spiritual perspective, but it is also important to note that you also can't achieve this only with a spiritual perspective while not fully embracing your physical being and the body that you inhabit currently. And might I suggest that if you are truly unhappy, begin to formulate a sincere goal to change that right away. Get very clear on who you are, what you are about, and what you want to be and begin to take steps to become exactly that. You have the power over your life. Don't let anyone else be the lead. Learn to love yourself fully and unconditionally so you can experience bliss in this world.

✿ TUNING INTO YOUR BODY WITH INTENTION

An activity that I like to do to honor my physical body is done in the shower. Take a little jar or bowl and mix sugar or sea salt with coconut, jojoba, olive, avocado, or grapeseed oil. You can add any of the essential oils listed in the chakra section of this chapter as well (you'll come to that section soon). While you are in the shower, use a washcloth to rub the salt or sugar mixture on each and every part of your skin in circular motions. Go slowly and work each nook and cranny of your skin.

As the dead skin cells are lifted away and the under skin begins to glow, pair this with intention. Out with anything that no longer serves your highest joys, and shine on the parts of yourself that were already there and waiting to be seen. Talk to your body in a way that matters. Especially as you go through this book and realize that each part of your body represents an emotional pattern, work with it as you address the physical. Give your body love. Absolutely no criticizing of your body. Only loving thoughts are permitted in this exercise.

Formulate your own affirmations as you scrub each part of your body. Go deeper and see if you find any area that has been stagnant with energy and rub it deeply and with intention to help anything that is stale. Rub up and down your body and see the salt or sugar all over your skin before you rinse it off. Then as you rinse off your body, collect anything you found that needs to go and talk to it and send it off with love down the drain forever.

The Mental/Emotional Body

All of the emotions that you currently experience, the stored emotions and even into past-life traumas, deal with how you digest your actions and the actions of others that have had a direct effect on you. Emotions are considered a conscious experience where you feel pain or pleasure and the realms in between the two. The emotional body and the mental body are one in the same to me. The mental process is centered on your emotions. The fight, flight, or freeze response is a direct reaction from both the emotional body and the physical body. This is solid mind/brain reaction. The mind is the emotions that brought on the need for a flight, fight, or freeze response and the body reaction is coming from the amygdala in the brain.

The central nervous system (governing the brain and spinal cord) connects into a space beyond the physical. It is in this space that the physical body and the emotional body collide. The term for the energetic spine is the sushumna. It is the storehouse for the chakras that we will be discussing later in this chapter. The emotional/mental body manifests itself through the physical body, the spiritual body, and the energy body. The emotions are what make us human. They are our feelers and our perceptions of those feelings. They can heal us or cause tremendous illness within our physical beings if not processed, accepted, and released.

The emotions explain how we feel in any given situation. There is an emotion wheel available to help you identify your feelings more easily. The emotional body is supercharged. It has such power and so much love if that is the tendency we have to lean toward. Or so much fear if that is the space we lean toward. Look at the emotion wheel to help yourself identify with your emotions and feelings within your body/mind as you go through this book and begin to practice self-healing.

Ways to nourish your emotional body are to become aware and expressive of your thoughts and feelings. Learning to be honest with yourself and the world around you is an awakening that can be painful if you let it. It will lead to great change to stop sparing your feelings or anyone else's. But there is a way to come into your own sacred truth where any form of lying just won't cut it anymore. That is such an incredible liberation and I want this for you. Work with yourself. Stop covering up for yourself or others. Be kind, be compassionate, be mindful, and be honest.

Come into a place where you own your actions and your words. Give that respect to you and to everyone around you. Clear the pains and shames that you have endured and stop any cycle if you have played a part in dishing them out to anyone else (including you). To enjoy your mental/emotional body you must own your space by living fully present in your body.

❀ CLEAR YOUR MIND

An activity to practice daily is to clear your mind. Part of the practice of meditation is done through simply allowing. When you sit down to meditate, don't think of it as meditating. Think of it as clearing your mind and emotional space. Sit or lie down. Close your eyes. Get acquainted with what the Buddhists refer to as the monkey mind. The monkey mind is that restless mind chatter that goes on all the time in your head, especially when you are trying to quiet it down.

Just hang out and watch your thoughts for a bit first. Let whatever wants to come in enter the mind, but you just watch it. No attachment. Don't judge it. Don't do the "what in the world are you talking about right now?" Learn to become friends with your monkey mind. Once you allow the monkey to chatter, it will naturally talk less. You cannot meet force with force on this one. You have to be the one to lay down, go neutral, and not attach yourself to any emotion that comes through your mind right now. Just become the observer. This doesn't even have to lead to some great meditation. It is simply the process of clearing your emotional space for a bit. No big release, no big *ahas*, nothing. Just simply being there and watching what is going on in that mind of yours is enough. It helps you to go deeper into yourself without doing all the extra work.

Do this often. Do it for a few minutes every day. Clear the space, watch your mental space, and don't judge it. Just be there. The results will come without so much thought.

Facing Our Pain

I went to a Native American medicine woman (shaman) for healing. It is believed in this tradition that when your heart is broken it actually is broken and that pieces of your soul do leave the body to reside elsewhere. Some parts of the soul sit on the other side with loved ones who left before us. I had a piece that left when my father died. I never told her that my dad died or what age I was when that happened. Yet, she brought back a soul piece of me at age thirteen and specifically told me that I was thirteen and with my dad when she found that piece of me. (I was, in fact, thirteen when he died suddenly.) It is the magic of what your body can tell someone who is trained to listen. She said that when she went to retrieve this soul piece of me, I looked at her and said, "Leave me alone, I'm with my dad." She had to get my dad to deliver that soul piece back to me because I couldn't bear to part with him again.

I was not at all prepared for what was to come after having soul pieces returned to me. For me, bringing back a piece of my soul that left because it was utterly traumatized was not easy at all. The soul piece was exactly how it was when it left me. It did not go sit on the other side and get all cleaned up and healed. Placing a traumatized piece of my soul back into me was utterly painful all over again. Had I known what I was really in for, I would have been much better prepared for this work and the work that comes after. It was a tremendous experience nonetheless, but I did not want to write this the way I've seen it so many other times, where the dark side of this process was not revealed ahead of time.

Energy is so much more than something clinical and so is the body. We are narrow in our vision. This shaman stunned me with her knowledge of my body and mind by talking directly to my energy centers. We did not have a conversation, she did not want me getting in the way of what my body had to tell her. After visiting the Upledger Institute, I learned that Dr. Upledger felt the same way. He did not want to know your story before he treated the body. He didn't want your information getting in the way of what your body had to say. In my own practice, I am open to hearing what my clients came to see me for and I allow them to share anything they want to share, but only once I've gotten started with the work. I also do not want to hear their story before we begin. The body is the messenger, if we know how to decipher its meanings.

In order to heal, no matter what sort of person or doctor you turn to for the healing, you must be willing to face the hardest days of your life, again. Then, hopefully, you can help those painful parts heal and integrate them back into your whole being. The goal is not to gloss over any of it. The goal is to face it, feel it, and then learn to integrate it, uniting the you that experienced the trauma with who you were before the trauma occurred. This allows a person to no longer identify with the trauma, but to learn from it and truly move beyond it. If you can do that, you will feel a happiness and fulfillment that you may not have felt since before any tragedy or trauma came across your life. This is the case in many healing arenas, not just shamanism. Pain must be faced head-on and acknowledged if it is to be conquered, and healing must be approached from multiple angles—not just from a physical angle but from an emotional angle as well. It is in our bodies that we can experience being *cured* of something. But it is within the spirit that we can be fully *healed*. Integrate all of the parts to complete the whole. The body, the mind/emotions, the spirit, and the energy inhabits it all. *You can change your life.*

No matter what you may have been through or where you are today, you have everything you need to change the path. The mind is so incredibly powerful that if you are under hypnosis and someone touches you with their bare finger and tells you that it is burning you, you very well may actually visibly blister. The mind in union with the body can heal in ways that no one to this point has ever allowed you to believe. It is all there inside you just waiting to come out and thrive. Make up your mind, seek and accept help from every place it is offered, and commit yourself fully to the goodness that is beyond anything you've experienced before. Miracles happen. Spontaneous healing has occurred more than mainstream stories tell. Intentional healing is my sincere hope for you.

The Energetic Body

The energy field of one's body is something that is beyond the physical dimension. There are three ways that a person's energy patterns can be accessed and understood. First is the aura—overlapping energy patterns that can be seen in a person's energy field. When someone sees the aura, they are usually able to see colors and other patterns that make up a field larger than the physical body. The aura changes with emotions and development. Through a person's aura, one can read where their energy is strongest and weakest. When you see the various colors that surround you, it's pretty amazing.

Another avenue into a person's energy body is through the meridian channels running through a person's body. These energetic pathways will be discussed several times throughout this book. The third way to access and understand the energy body is through the chakra system of the body.

The Chakras

The chakras give us another way to both understand and heal the body on a physical, emotional, energetic, and spiritual level. The chakras (pronounced SHAK-rahs or CHAK-rahs) are your body's energy centers that negotiate both physical and subtle energies. Each chakra is associated with a specific area of the body. The body has seven chakras. These are the main energy centers in the body that store emotions. When we say things like "he/she broke my heart," we know instinctively that we are talking about the heart chakra, the energetic heart. We know that we are not discussing the actual pericardium. We have always known the heart as two specific entities: as the emotional part of ourselves but also as a specific organ in the body with four chambers.

In truth, there are several hundred chakras throughout the body, but there are seven main ones that we focus on. The seven main chakras govern the places of energetic consciousness, and they each correlate to both the actual spine and the nerve plexus in the physical body. The chakras are vital to our overall health and well-being, and to dismiss this would be detrimental to both. Each chakra represents a state of consciousness and each one has a specific feeling and tone.

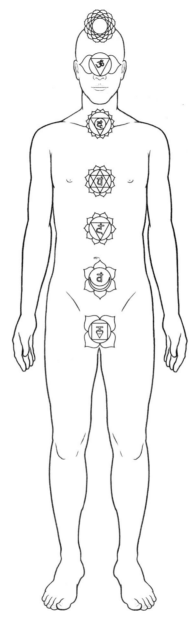

The Seven Main Chakras

First Chakra—Root Chakra

The first chakra, known as the root chakra, is located at the base of the spinal column and corresponds to the sacral plexus. The authentic name for this chakra is the *Muladhara*. The color is red. The sound associated with this chakra is Lam, and it has four petals. This chakra governs the connection to the earth and earthly materials. This includes things that are material possessions. Influence, fame, and fortune resonate with this chakra.

First Chakra Stones:
Ruby (red) red jasper and black tourmaline

First Chakra Essential Oils:[1]
Vetivert has an earthy aroma. It is a calming and grounding oil that helps one to feel rooted in the physical body. In this way, it can help one to feel present and empowered. It is an oil of choice for those who want to feel connected to nature and nature spirits.

Cedarwood is relaxing and clarifying due to its high levels of sesquiterpenes. It promotes a feeling of security and safety to feel open to creating connections, or "roots," within one's social communities and environment.

Patchouli is grounding and stabilizing, connecting one to the physical body. It has the ability to diffuse anger, soothe anxiety, and enhance feelings of peace.

Black pepper is a stimulating oil that can anchor the self and assist in releasing negative emotions and behaviors, such as self-judgment, to reclaim self-empowerment.

---

1. Essential Oils for this section provided by Stephanie Colletti of www.witchymamawisdom.com.

Second Chakra—Sacral Chakra

The second chakra, known as the soul chakra, is located around the reproductive organs/ genital area and corresponds to the prostate plexus. The authentic name for this chakra is *Swadhisthana*. The element associated with the chakra is water. The color associated in this area is orange. It governs creativity and sexual energy. The sound associated with this chakra is Vam, and it has six petals.

Second Chakra Stones:

Citrine, (orange) carnelian, orange calcite

Second Chakra Essential Oils:

Orange is known as an oil of abundance. It is uplifting and encouraging, and it inspires creativity.

Sandalwood is calming and sensual. Known to be an aphrodisiac, it can ignite passions.

Ylang Ylang has a soft, intoxicating floral scent. It can promote feelings of sensuality, balance, and joy.

Bergamot can assist one to be "in the flow" of life. It cleanses negative energy and replaces feelings of hope and optimism. Do not put bergamot directly on the skin.

Third Chakra—Solar Plexus Chakra

The third chakra, at the navel, corresponds to the solar plexus. The authentic name for this chakra is *Manipura*. The color associated with this is yellow. This chakra governs trust in self and honoring your own instincts. When you feel something in your gut, it is the solar plexus chakra activating. The element associated with this is fire. The sound associated with this chakra is Ram, and it has ten petals.

Third Chakra Stones:

Yellow topaz and (yellow) citrine

Third Chakra Essential Oils:

Lemon uplifts spirits and reduces mental fatigue through increased focus and clarity of thought.

Grapefruit is energizing and encourages a positive relationship with the physical body.

Helichrysum can aid victims of trauma to overcome adversity while building a sense of courage and strength.

Juniper is associated with the element of fire, purifying and cleansing to promote confidence and courage.

Fourth Chakra—Heart Chakra

The fourth chakra is located at the heart. The authentic name for this chakra is *Anahata*. The color associated with this area is green—the color associated with healing. The heart chakra correlates directly to the cardiac plexus. This governs your ability to love and be loved. The element associated with this chakra is ether. The sound associated with this is Yam, and it has twelve petals.

The first four chakras of the body are considered to govern your earth self, which is why they have earth elements governing each chakra. The remaining three chakras enter into your spiritual space, and therefore are not governed by elements. Once the first four chakras are opened, then you can start to experience the joy of the following chakras.

Fourth Chakra Stones:

Emerald (green), rose quartz (pink), green aventurine

Fourth Chakra Essential Oils:

Rose is a high vibrational oil that gently opens the heart to unconditional peace, love, and acceptance.

Lavender has an intoxicating floral scent that is soothing, calming, and relaxing to the mind and body.

Geranium is healing to the heart and inspires us to continue to live with an open heart regardless of past pain.

Eucalyptus has the ability to open and cleanse the heart space on physical and emotional levels.

Fifth Chakra—Throat Chakra

The fifth chakra is located at the throat and corresponds to the laryngeal plexus. The color associated with this is blue. The throat chakra governs your ability to be heard as well as to speak your truth. When we do not speak honestly or from a loving manner, our throat chakra becomes blocked, resulting in sore throats or other issues in our throat. The authentic name for this chakra is *Vishuddha*. It is associated with the sound Hum, and it has sixteen petals.

Fifth Chakra Stones:

Sapphire (dark) or aquamarine (light) turquoise, blue lace agate

Fifth Chakra Essential Oils:

Rosemary has an earthy, herbaceous aroma that is uplifting to the mind and enhances communication of truth.

Cypress is a stimulating oil that encourages feelings of flexibility and to trust in the flow of life.

Jasmine has a sweet floral aroma that promotes clear communication, which can enhance intimate relationships.

Marjoram is a warm, spicy oil that can open the heart and transform negative life experiences into positive self-empowerment.

Sixth Chakra—Third Eye Chakra

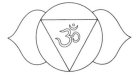

The sixth chakra is the third eye chakra, located between the eyebrows and slightly up. This corresponds directly to the cavernous plexus. The color associated with this is indigo. The authentic name for this chakra is the *Ajna* chakra. It corresponds to the sound *om*. It has two petals. This is the place where we are more able to see into the spiritual realm. Often referred to as our spiritual center.

Sixth Chakra Stones:

Amethyst (purple) or chevron amethyst (various shades of purple and white) azurite, lapis lazuli

Sixth Chakra Essential Oils:

Palo Santo is derived from Palo Santo "Holy Wood" and used to cleanse and purify negativity.

Thyme is a stimulating heart opener that teaches us to live in the present.

Lemongrass is a soft, grassy citrus scent that assists in healing and inspires the optimism and courage to move forward.

Hyssop has a soft, woody aroma that is spiritually cleansing and meditative.

Seventh Chakra—Crown Chakra

The seventh chakra, known as the crown chakra, is located at the top of the head and beyond. This is the spiritual reason behind a baby's soft spot. It is the last place to close when we come to earth, as it is our connection to the heavens. The authentic name for this is the *Sahasrara* chakra.

The sound associated with the chakra is also *om*. This chakra does not have petals, as once this chakra has been opened all of the petals from the previous chakras are turned upward and create the perfect number fifty that represents the fifty petals that create a lotus flower. A picture of the flower at the top of the head would look like a circle, with fifty petals expanding out over the skull. In opening all of the chakras, the lotus petals go from facing down to turning upward toward the sky. This activates and opens the kundalini shakti.

Seventh Chakra Stones:

Clear quartz, diamond (white/clear), white topaz

Seventh Chakra Essential Oils:

Frankincense has a warm, sweet, woody smell that is calming, centering, and spiritually expansive.

Myrrh has a warm, earthy scent that is emotionally supportive with the ability to assist in deepening spiritual connection.

Tea tree has an earthy aroma and is known to be mentally and emotionally purifying.

Angelica opens spiritual connection, communication, and guidance through Divine union.

❀ CHAKRA CLEANSING MEDITATION [2]

Cleansing your chakras will set a good foundation for overall healing of the body on both energetic and emotional levels. Lie down on your back and get comfortable. Let your feet fall out to each side and bring your arms out to the sides, allowing your hands to open freely. Breathe in a long, deep breath and hold it for a moment. With your breath held, sense a wave of energy down your body from the crown of your head to the soles of your feet. Anyplace within your body that you feel blocked, sad, stressed, stagnant, or darkness in color, notice it and gather it up. With a gust in your exhale, push it all down and out through the feet.

Repeat this pattern with each breath—in, hold and release, and push through. Begin to feel the energy of your body. What is open, what is not. What is joyful, what is not. Create the rainbow within. Red is at the base of your spine, top of the

---

2. To listen to Emily guide you through this meditation, please go to her website (emilyafrancisbooks.com) and click on CDs. You will find this meditation offered for free.

legs. Imagine a red ruby over this area and anyplace in that red ruby that is not sparkling and shining light like a ruby gemstone, allow the dark specs to fall away as you feel your breath and your intention clean it entirely. Envision your higher self massaging and cleaning the stones above each chakra. With your intention, allow the darkness that might be in this area or on your stone to fall away gently and with ease.

Once you see the red ruby over this space become shiny and new, move upward to the second chakra of orange just below the navel. Imagine the eternity symbol (a figure eight) circling through the front of your body to the back of your body just below the navel and in the lower back. See the color orange like a citrine just over this area. Notice if there are any dark specks in your crystal. Allow the darkness to fall away as you shine your light and open up your creative joys in this area and let the energy flow through that eternity symbol back and forth, front and back.

When the citrine is shiny and new, move upward to the third chakra, the solar plexus chakra. Now just above your navel see the color yellow as a yellow topaz above your navel and below your ribs, also to the back of the body. See in your mind this beautiful gemstone and notice again if there is any darkness attached to this stone. This represents your trust of self and your inner knowingness. When you know something in your gut, it is your truth. Hold on tight to that feeling and trust it always. Notice if there are any dark spots on your yellow topaz and allow the darkness to fall away with your breath and with your intention.

Move upward into the fourth chakra and see a green emerald just above your heart. You may also decide to use a pink rose quartz for unconditional love along with the emerald or by itself. That is entirely up to you and your interpretation of what you see within your own heart space. Notice this amazing color of green and play with it in your mind. Your heart chakra is the doorway to your soul and your heart. This governs your ability to love and be loved. If you see any dark specks in your emerald, I ask that you allow that darkness to again fall away, using your breath and your intention. Let the emerald become lighter, shiny, and bright. Breathe into this sacred stone and give thanks for the love you have to share with yourself and with others and the love you are now able to receive from yourself as well as from others. Clear the cobwebs to your soul in this space and let love in.

Move up into the fifth chakra and see above your throat a beautiful sapphire blue or a light blue of aquamarine, depending again on what you see within yourself. Look deeply into the stone that you have chosen to represent your throat area. See if there are variants of blues in this stone. Some light, some dark, and some shiny, and again notice any specs of darkness or drab, stagnant energy that might be within this powerful stone. This governs your ability to speak your truth and do it kindly. Allow yourself to be heard and speak with intention of clarity and not to harm, but never to cower from your own honesty of where you are in any given moment. Use your breath and your intention to let this stone clear and clean in the most glorious way. You always deserve to be heard, to speak up, to be honest, and not come from a space of anger or rage. Learning to speak with honesty and clarity with intention breaks the rage patterns. Go into this new level of communication with comfort and ease as you become more assertive.

Move up into the third eye chakra and see the color amethyst. You may also see several purple colors and white, which would indicate that for you a chevron amethyst is a better choice for this chakra. Look into this beautiful purple color. This is the area where spirit can come in. This is the area that you come into a higher space of consciousness. If your third eye is slightly opened or even closed, go within and ask spirit to help you open this area of your being at a pace that is healthy for you. See the purple stone clean and shine as any darkness falls away, and you are able to see more clearly and from a deeper and higher space.

Move up into the crown chakra now. Even though the color for this is violet, I prefer to use a clear quartz or a diamond. This is the presence of all light now creating this great, white light above your head. This is the area that is the last to close when we come to earth because it is our connection to the heavens. Allow this shining, beautiful, radiant light to open your crown chakra and feel your own connections coming back in without fear, without hesitation, and with complete trust that you are safe and protected. Use your breath and your intention to clear this space and the stone that you choose to represent your own sacred energy.

Now swirling above you and within you are the colors of the rainbow and the colors of your body energies swirling together: red, orange, yellow, green, blue, indigo, and violet. They are now meshing into one solid white light of purity, kindness, and love of the greatest magnitude. Stay in this orb of white light for as long as you are able. Let the great white light clean every part of your being. Be open to this healing experience and stay in it as long as you are able and present.

When you are ready to come out, slowly begin to wiggle your fingers and toes. Keep your eyes closed until the very end. Roll to your right side (unless you are pregnant, in which case roll to your left). Stay on your right side for a few breaths and then place the left palm flat on the floor in front of your face. Still keeping your eyes closed, push off up and help yourself come to a seated position. Sit up, eyes closed, spine straight, and legs crossed comfortably. Breathe into this space. Let the energy of this meditation spread itself into every cell of your being and be absorbed into the muscle memory. This way you can come back to this space more easily. As you slowly come out of this meditation, try to stay inside the light. Keep the light in you and around you as much as you are able. When you are ready, open your eyes and come back to center. Return to this meditation often.

Chapter 3

Emotional Release
and Energy Work

Being able to help people experience emotional release is my special gift. It isn't something I advertise or offer as any part of regular conversation, nor do I promote this work. People find me when they are meant to find me for this specific purpose. People who have been clients of mine for years never know I can do this work until one day something is wrong either physically, spiritually, emotionally, or energetically, and we change up what we've been doing for the years before. I take this subject very seriously and consider it my most sacred work.

While emotional release isn't something that I can teach you how to do step-by-step (it just doesn't work that way!), I can share some of the finer details, methods, and nuances of the process so that you can get a deeper look into the healing practices used by professional bodyworkers. What I can do here is explain some of the energy techniques used in such work as well as experiences that I've had and been witness to. Not all bodyworkers facilitate emotional releases, and not all bodywork is the same. Some practitioners utilize Reiki and some are trained in the Healing Touch Program™. Some practitioners utilize clinical massage techniques. Some practitioners utilize what they generically call "energy work." Everyone has a unique perspective, and learning more about different healing methods is beneficial from both the standpoint of a student who is learning to become a massage therapist or other bodyworker, as well as for the person receiving such treatments who wants to know more about exactly what is being done to their body and why. Here are some of the techniques that I use in my own healing practice.

Energy Work

Energy work is an umbrella term describing a number of different techniques used to help the body heal itself through touch and through intuitive contact with the energies of the body. Energy work can be practiced by massage therapists, Reiki practitioners, Healing Touch™ practitioners, as well as people who have had no formal training but have a true and honest desire to help someone to heal. Energy work is what is referred to in the Bible as "the laying of hands," and Reiki is simply another technique and school of thought surrounding energy work. Basically it all amounts to the same. Your hands are placed on or near a person's body, and we open ourselves to be a clear conduit for unconditional love and healing energy. Whenever I do energy work of any type, no matter what I call it, I know that I am opening to the highest light and positive energy of the Divine. And so does any person or animal who receives from me.

I have a friend who learned energy work from a teacher who describes it as "removing the layers in the energy field." We start at the surface, asking "What is hurting?" and "What do you feel?" Can we "see" anything if we close our eyes, hold our hands above the body, and do a body scan? Do we see any images or colors, or do any areas seem particularly hot or cold? If we do feel any changes in temperature, can we turn it into something tangible? Are there any painful memories or emotions being stored here? And if so, can we remove them for the person by visualizing and doing things like turning that emotional energy into a ball and rolling it away, putting it into a box and shutting the top, then moving the box out of the mind or throwing it into the garbage or into a river? You do all that for the top layer of energy, then you go a layer deeper and do the exact same thing, and again deeper, until we basically hit the bone. There are no more layers, we have gone as deep as we can to help them uncover what is really happening and how we can help them remove it for themselves.

Everyone approaches energy work differently. I liked hearing my friend's way of working. It's interesting and helpful. I find in many cases people all over the place discussing energy work like it's a sacred science that has so many rules and applications. I felt for a long time that I must not know nearly as much as they do because I don't talk like that. I don't know how to put rules of order into this work, I simply clear the space, ask for spiritual help and guidance, and then trust my hands and my gut. My approach is pretty straightforward and simple—I just trust the process and am open to whatever may come up.

I had a partner with whom I would practice and attune people to Reiki. I never realized it until she pointed out to people in the class that she is very methodical and I am very organic. She said that she reads the book and goes in the exact order that the book tells her to do. She rarely if ever deviates from instruction. She said that I read the book and then I throw it out and do my own thing. I'm not sure I have ever heard a better compliment about myself! I had never thought about myself in this manner before that day, and I liked it very much. So while you might be very methodical and by the book yourself, I do encourage you to go deeper and let the body tell you what it wants you to know. Don't use this book as anything more than a tool for gaining a deeper understanding of the body and its emotions. This information is to help you heal yourself and anyone else who may need you—but there is no order to it, just a straight up offering from many amazing people who helped me put it into words.

Creating a Sacred Space

Placing your hands on someone carries with it great responsibility. Whenever I'm going to be doing energy work, I like to prepare myself as well as the client and the space before we begin. To prepare myself, I practice self-cleaning techniques and I connect to the highest energy source through prayer. I smudge myself with sage to help purify my energies and raise my vibration, and I also waft the smoldering herb bundle around the space we'll be in so that the aromatic, cleansing smoke reaches the ceiling, the floors, and each of the four corners of the room.

Then, I use the sage to help prepare the client for the work, as well. I take them outside, and I wave the sage so that the smoke circles and swirls around the entire person. I have them stand still with their feet apart and their arms out to the sides. I wave the smoke stick down and around each arm, around their hands, up and down the center line and the throat, around their head, and down and around their legs. I have them lift their feet and I carefully swirl the smoke under each foot. I then tell them to turn around and I do the same to the entire back side of them. I sometimes slap the smudge stick forward to get more smoke into a certain area.

The client and myself both prepared, attention is turned back to the space in which we will be doing the energy work. State your intention over and over in your mind or out loud as you waft the fragrant smoke around the space. Sage is believed to drive out any negative energy. Some people like to burn sweet grass at the same time or after burning sage, as it is believed to bring in positive healing energy. The smoke from burning sage has been proven to help clean the air of bacteria[3], but if you prefer, you can instead mix a few drops of sage essential oil in a glass spray bottle with some water, and use this to spritz your body or the room.

A sacred space helps facilitate energy work and emotional release of any kind. In order for a space to be sacred, you must create it to be that way. There are a number of ways to do this, and there is no such thing as one right way to do it, as everyone has their own preferred methods of creating a sacred space. For me, I put my fingers up and circle them to the ceiling as I repeat the words my teacher taught me: "I cast a circle around this space that only the highest light may enter." Then I will draw certain Reiki symbols in the corners of the walls and on the main walls with my hand. I let the person on the massage table know that I am about to pray and set the tone of the space. I ask them if they would prefer for me to pray out loud or silently. I then open up with prayer, inviting all of my spirit helpers in. I also ask them if they would like to pray and who they would like to invite into our sacred space. I offer this to them because they should have every say in who comes in and who does not. They also might want to hear that they are in fact in a safe space, and I am setting our intentions for the session clearly and in a powerful and safe way. I like to include things such as, "If it is your will, please heal all involved" or "Please help lead us to the greatest good and highest joy of this person."

Items to Help Create Your Own Sacred Space

There are several ways that you can make a beautiful, safe space to invoke healing energy. Some of them include:

---

3. Brandon Richard, "Study: Burning Sage (smudging) Can Eliminate Harmful Air Pollutants," accessed May 8, 2017 at http://www.davidwolfe.com/burning-sage-smudging/?c=pwf&vp=dchop.

Sea Salt: An excellent protector and energy cleanser. I keep a bowl of sea salt in my practice room, and I rub a pinch between my hands so that I can clear myself of the energy of the person I've just been treating. You can place salt in any room to help protect the space and to help clear it of negative energy, or sprinkle it on any person (including yourself!) to help purify their energies. To strengthen the effect, mix the salt with holy water and sprinkle it down the spine, on the crown of the head, or on the palms of the hands or soles of the feet. Sea salt is also wonderful for a detox bath to help release impurities from the body. (See appendix A for bath recipes.)

Mirrors: Incredible and real deflectors. When facilitating for someone else, just have a one-sided mirror pointing away from your chest to protect you from any unwanted energy coming at you. It is super powerful. You can imagine a mirror or really wear a mirror. Both work.

The White Cloak: Imagine yourself stepping into a white-light cloak all around you as you enter this space and work on someone. You must always keep your person protected, but you also must keep yourself protected. You don't know what that person will be laying down and you do not need to absorb it. Stay inside your white-light cloak at all times.

Crystals and Pendants: Wearing stones will protect you. An easy one to start with is a simple clear quartz. This helps transmute energies and keep you protected. Smokey quartz helps to dispel negative energy. A lot of energy workers will be sure to have a smokey quartz on them somewhere if not around the neck. Wearing a rose quartz near your heart is wonderfully blissful, as it is a stone of unconditional love. Some people buy necklaces that are specifically for protection or an increase in energy or for whatever specific intention the necklace has been designed with. I also like to use apophyllite stones at the head and foot of the table to keep my energy and the recipient's energy separate. Having two of these stones is very important to me while engaging in this work. We will discuss stones further in appendix A.

Hand Placement

After the space, myself, and the client are prepared, it's time to begin the actual energy work. I like to start in the safest places—the feet, head, or shoulders. I usually go with the feet, as most people don't get nervous when you touch this area. I put both of my hands on the soles of the person's feet to help them to feel more grounded (if they are lying facedown (prone) or I place my hands on the tops of their feet if they are lying faceup (supine). I can feel the swirls of energy through their entire body from just the feet. I close my eyes and feel the pulse—first the actual pulse of the blood flow and then the energy pulses. Some of the energy pulses seem to swirl around in long circles, while others are short and wiry. Some have a distinct path, and some are fragmented. All these varying energy pulses combine together as a giant, circling loop of full body sensations.

After the feet, I usually will place my hands over the person's knees, then I may go for my favorite place—the heart and solar plexus. If they aren't ready for that, I'll first place my hands under their head and then move on to the shoulders. It's really about your and the person's comfort levels. Once I get past the basics and the client is more receptive and relaxed, I do tend to spend a longer time in that main area of the body, placing my left hand on the high chest (above the breasts) and my right hand just above the navel. This helps the person to bring balance to the solar plexus and the heart space. I like to say to them, "Imagine there is a rainbow of energy and love connecting from one hand to the other, but circling inside your own body. Feel the chest and solar plexus aligning." This hand positioning and visualization is very helpful to do whenever a person is feeling off-balance. You can always come back to this center. There are many books specifically on Reiki or energy work that will offer a step-by-step protocol of hand placements in a particular order. As I said before, I do not follow a standard protocol and therefore do not offer it in this book.

If the person I'm working on is laying facedown, I like to place my hands over those same spots on the back, corresponding to the location of the solar plexus and heart space. I place one hand on the mid upper back and the other on the middle and then lower back while keeping my upper hand at the heart space. The back side of the body is much less guarded than the front side is. Because the front side is so guarded, however, it is also more vulnerable and may be able to release well having hands in those areas. Keep in mind that we are among the few species on the planet that walk around with our most valuable and vulnerable organs exposed to the world. Most walk on all fours and their heart, lungs, stomach, intestines, and liver are hidden from straight contact. We humans have them right up and out in the open. This is very sensitive, and we need to remember this and respect this aspect of our bodies.

In my experience, knowing that the back side does not have the armor that the front side does, I believe that having the hand placements on the front side encourages a deeper release of emotions, while having my hands on the back side of their body allows me to help replenish the release with loving, healing energy. Whatever yucky stuff went out, we replace with something so much cleaner. I hold my hands on each body area for about three minutes at a time (which is the recommended time in Reiki practice) as I send a flow of pure, loving energy into their body, then I'll move my hands to a different area and do the same. If there is a place on their body that needs you to stay longer, stay until you are led to move your hands to the next place that you are called to. If I'm working on a baby or an animal, I lessen the time to about a quarter of the usual and I also lessen the flow of energy that I'm directing into them so that it's not too overwhelming. Babies and animals are much more sensitive, so it doesn't have to be as intense.

What I usually do is begin with the client faceup (supine), then end with the client facedown (prone). This way, if they have not yet released by the latter half of the session and they want to, they might be more encouraged to do so in the facedown position. When a person is facedown, they may be more open to allowing themselves to cry, since they know I can't see their face. It's sort of a darker space and feels more private to them. When they are facedown, they talk less and so do I. It's a different energy to release from. For many, this is the preferred position for letting go.

Breathing

One simple technique that can lead to intense results is to utilize the breath to help guide emotional energy out of the body. I begin by setting the tone with my own deeper breathing, exhaling audibly so that the client will hear it. Soon, their breathing patterns begin to match. I ask them as they inhale to feel whatever sensations are coming through them, and on the exhale, to send the feelings and emotions down the length of their body to exit through the soles of their feet. I tell them to hold their breath and feel the pain for a moment, then blow out hard from an open mouth. Each breath should be intense, audible, and meaningful. Breathing in this manner can open the gateway to an emotional release.

When I'm leading the client through the breathing, I find it helpful to place my hands on the top of their head. As the person breathes and pushes the release through, I will also exhale loudly and deeply right into the crown of their head, assisting with their own breath to help move all that stale emotional energy out of the body. I will inhale and hold the breath for a moment, and wait for the client to do the big exhale, or if they need some prompting, I go ahead and lead them through example to do the big exhale. Then with a giant gusto, I exhale *through them* through the head, imagining my breath flowing all the way down the length of their body to send all that unwanted energy out through the soles of their feet. I keep my hands flat to the top of the person's head, making a diamond shape with my thumbs and index fingers, and I breathe deeply into that space that I have made just over the crown chakra. It is my job as the facilitator to help the person get their emotional stuff out. It is my job to watch their body and their face as things begin to move. The breath is always a huge platform from which to begin the bigger releases.

Coughing

Often, deep breathing will lead to coughing. Coughing is a wonderful way to release emotions from the body. It helps clear the throat chakra of any energy blockages, and it also helps to let out feelings that are buried down deep. Remember, the throat chakra governs your ability to speak your truth. When you begin to cough out some of that pain, times in your life when you either weren't heard or never spoke up are coming forward. I encourage the person to let out their feelings with the cough. I let them know this is a healthy sign of release, and to keep doing it. If they begin to bend over to really get the cough moving, I do whatever I can to assist them. I hold their back or shoulders if it feels right to do so. I do whatever is needed to be the backbone for the person as they face their sadness and times of shame. I tell them to let it all come out. As they cough more and more, this usually leads to tears and, again, to a deeper release.

Crying

Tears are the number one most effective way to release serious, deep pains. Tears are the physical manifestation of pain leaving the body. Once they're out, you cannot put them back in. It is the years of pain and shame, guilt, fear, exhaustion—you name it—leaving the body for good. Once the tears come, it's best to encourage them to keep on coming. When a client starts crying as part of the release process, I become a little more vocal and encouraging. It takes courage to become so vulnerable, and I need them to know it is completely safe to do so. I encourage them by letting them know that they are in a safe space and that I am there simply to help them release. There is no judgment here in this healing space, and we will not discuss this following the treatment session unless they specifically want to and ask to do so. This is their own sacred time and things like this don't happen often. And they don't happen time and time again, either. Emotional releases are intense, and those grand, soul-shaking, life-changing releases may only happen once or twice in a lifetime.

Going with the Flow

When the tears start to flow, that's when I slow down any movements of my hands and lighten up the touch. This doesn't mean I get lazy and just stand there or give an idle, one-handed massage. It means I simply slow down and lessen the pressure so that the energy can be coaxed to flow out more freely. I notice that when I feel the energy becoming intense, I have a habit (and I don't at all think I'm alone in this) to add pressure to my touch because I want the energy to be felt more or something. I have to remind myself to keep the thumb in with the other fingers, and place my hands so that the mid-palm where the energy is strongest can easily come through. I also have to loosen all my joints, so that nothing is straightened out and blocking the flow of the energy from leaving my hands.

When we get rigid, the energy can block in our wrists, knees, ankles, elbows, or shoulders and not fully make its way into the client. You must be willing to flow with the energy and not try to push it through. You must trust that it is moving and happening and slow it down, opening yourself and your body up to the process so that the person receiving the energy gets all that is designed to go to them. This is also the case when I'm applying pressure during a massage. If I loosen up and let the power and energy flow through me, I'm able to go much deeper. I am always reminding myself to back off and let the flow of energy do its work. I try to be gentle with myself as well as with the person I'm working on, and this means that I must work *with* the flow, and not against it. I try to be an open channel to the person I'm treating as well as to the higher powers (I like to think of it as God or Great Spirit). I keep myself out of it. I do not offer stories of anything in my own life, and I don't offer advice or opinions. I simply stay with them, I keep my hands on them, and I keep setting the tone with the breath.

Focus and Awareness

I also try to tap into my client and hear what words or songs come into my mind. When I am working, spirit communicates with me through playing different songs in my head as I work. The songs change like a radio station when my hands are on someone, or even if I am meeting someone new. Songs that are not my own, that I wouldn't think about come up. So, I do my best to listen to the lyrics to get a gauge on where the person is at that given time. As I move my hands, the songs change. This is one way that spirit works with me to keep me tuned into the person.

From there, I may approach the person with some information or I might create a mantra that I repeat over and over again for them in my head. Each person is different to me, so I do not carry one specific mantra to repeat. If I were to choose something generic, it would be something along the lines of "Pure love and healing energy comes to you now. Prayers to you for peace and health." I repeat this over and over again during the session, uttering it silently within my mind and sometimes speaking it out loud. This keeps me present to the person and to the process, and it allows the energy to flow through me so that I can give to them as much as I can without my monkey mind ruining it for any of us. Some Buddhists use the term *monkey mind* to refer to all of those super animated thoughts that are scattered all over the place. I want to be in single-pointed focus for the person I'm working on, and I find that repeating an affirmation or mantra for the person's health and healing ensures that I am present and focused.

Mindfulness

I open my eyes often to scan the client's entire body throughout this process. My role is to be mindful of the person's body so that when a release comes up, I can take charge of the physical body as they focus on the emotional aspect. They don't have to think about their physical body anymore—I got it. They just need to focus their breath and thoughts to whatever it is that is pushing through and trying desperately to make its way out. People tend to try to fight and hide away the pains that are struggling to come out into the light. As the painful energy begins to move, it often will tuck itself away in some other part of the body. I remain watchful and mindful throughout the treatment session so that I can follow those pains wherever they go and ensure they make their way completely out. If I see the client wiggle, change positions, tuck their butt under, or crinkle their toes, I know there is energy on the move that is looking for a new hideout. Then it's up to me to play Sherlock Holmes and track it down. The muscles themselves provide clues as to what sort of emotional energy it is that I am dealing with.

The emotional truths that don't require real charting are these: Every person in some capacity in their lives feels under appreciated. Every person in their lives feels *less than* at times. Insecurities are for everyone. And problems in one's sex life are extremely common. *Everyone* has been through *something*! Everyone has had a loss, a devastating breakup, and many more things. Many have survived being handled inappropriately. The truth is, it's not for me to chase down and find out, it's for me to chase down and *get it out*. I don't need to know why the emotional energy became trapped in the muscle and I don't need to understand the exact nature of it, I just need to find it and help it find its way out of the client's body. I handle each person with care and I give them the space and safety to discuss whatever they want to discuss. I don't make assumptions and I don't lead the conversation. I just listen to the feelings moving through their body, and if they choose to share their feelings with me out loud, I try to validate that what they feel is understandable. I don't ask for details, as it shouldn't be an actual discussion. I simply say things like "How does this make you feel?" or "I'm sorry you're feeling that way." I keep my focus on maintaining that safe, sacred space in which to release, and I don't get nosy by letting curiosity get the better of me. It's for them to talk and for me to listen.

One question I absolutely never ask is "What happened?" This is a safe space for a person who is already vulnerable, and asking questions that are straight on puts them into a position of feeling like they have to tell you something that they might not want to tell. It also puts them in a position to feel like they should defend themselves or justify anything that comes up. I say things such as "Do you want to talk about it? Or do you want to simply go over it in your own mind and not say anything out loud? Both are fine. You do what you feel most comfortable with." In that way, I can encourage the person to face whatever it is, feel it, and let it release out of the body. Trust is essential. I remain mindful of what I'm saying and, unless there are certain images or strong feelings coming to me that I feel can help the situation, I generally speak very little as I work, unless they are someone who needs guiding.

In this sacred space and time, I do not think of myself at all. I am merely the facilitator and an open conduit through which spirit can guide my hands and my head. As the energy continues to flow through my hands, emotions that have been stored and held captive within the body begin to flow out as well. Emotional releases don't always happen, but when they do happen, the effects are truly transformative. Sometimes, the release of emotions can be an incredibly powerful and life-changing experience.

Emotional Release

Many years ago, I worked at a premiere medical spa mostly known for the celebrity clientele. I had a woman come to me who said that she had been to every doctor, massage therapist, chiropractor, and anything you can think of, and no one had ever been able to get rid of her constant pain behind her right shoulder blade. She basically challenged me to see if I had any "game." I tore at it and worked like a beast. I broke a sweat doing everything in my arsenal I knew to get this muscle to let go. I finally looked up at her, sweaty faced, and said, "This isn't physical. It's emotional." I asked her if she was familiar with Reiki, and would she be alright if we tried that as our next option. She said she had heard of it, had not ever received it, and that yes, she would be more than open to it. She is the only person I've ever put into a physically compromising position to do the energy work.

Generally, as I've said above, it is important to lighten up and go slower when adding in this component. But I knew with this woman, I would only get the results if I put her in a slight amount of discomfort. I put her right hand behind her back and put my knee up on the table against her bent arm to keep her hand right in that space. It was not pleasant for her, but it was necessary. I can't explain it, I just knew this was the way. I then opened my palms and began my prayers and running the energy. She got frustrated right out of the gate—which was my sign that she was about to release. People always get fidgety and slightly bothered just before the emotions come up, first in smaller spurts to bigger bubbles to almost steam coming out of the pores. I did ask her what was going through her head in that moment—not to think about it, not to analyze it, but just say it, blurt it out. She said something about how she was cheated on by someone she loved very much, but that it had happened years ago, way back when she was in high school. She found it bizarre to be thinking of something so long ago that meant nothing to her now. I kept her straight to the path of thought and guided her not to get off course by analyzing it. That could come later. Right now, I told her to stay present to the pain and present to the thoughts that were coming in. Suddenly, out of nowhere, we both heard this audible bubble pop, and the entire area completely softened and released in a way that was completely and utterly profound to us both. It was gone. That knot, pain, or whatever you want to label it that had sat just next to her shoulder blade in her back for so many years was no more. We had removed the energetic knife stab that had been laid there back in high school (this woman was easily in her sixties), and it was gone. She got up a new woman. We hugged tightly, aware that we had just connected ourselves to each other forever through the bond of this sacred and amazing experience. She was so tearful and grateful.

I share this story because there is more to it. At this particular spa, people eat together in large groups. This woman stood up and announced at the following meal that I had performed a *miracle* on her and told them all about her special encounter. The following day, people were scrambling in line to change their massage appointments to come to me for an emotional release. Each person who comes to this spa has a coordinator who calls them months in advance to get their desired daily treatments scheduled—you cannot just decide on the spur of the moment that you want to go to this new girl who does this emotional energy stuff!

The point here is that you cannot ever schedule an emotional release. It does not, will not, and cannot ever be something that you have decided in your basic conscious mind that you need and want. It won't ever happen.

When I say this, I am referring to *the* emotional release. There can be many emotional releases, and you can sign up for that if you are going through something. When my dog, who was the love of my life, got sick, I called my fellow massage therapist and asked her to work on me while I cried and released. That too is an emotional release. However, the one that I'm referring to really only happens once to a person. It is the beginning of a very new way of healing and tuning into your body and the way it holds memories. If you are lucky, you experience this massive connecting to your body in a deep and profound way, while crying your eyes out and unlocking those old pains and angers forever. You leave the session completely and utterly exhausted. You can barely function the rest of the day. You may continue to cry. You fall into bed unable to do anything else. And then you wake up completely renewed and ready for a new start. Those only happen once. The ones to follow are sweet little mini releases and yes, you can even schedule them ahead of time on occasion, depending on what you are dealing with. Someone in the midst of a divorce can easily call up and know ahead of time that they might cry while they are on the table. Someone who is very ill and facing a life-changing illness, they might be able to know ahead of time that they will cry. They might not realize that particular cry just might change it all.

Techniques for Emotional Release on Yourself

Energy work is not just something that you can facilitate for other people. I highly encourage you to explore doing this sacred work on yourself. You are fully capable of taking yourself to a deeper level of awareness and understanding of the pains you've hidden as well. No one knows your body or your life the way you do. Create a space within yourself to unveil complete honesty with your mind and your body. Below is a list of suggestions to help yourself release old patterns and pains.

Touch with Intention

The mind becomes involved with the body and the connection strengthens as soon as there is touch involved. Touch is the physical response that sets off brain wave activity and also creates the thought processes that stimulate the mind, therefore uniting your body-mind. I like to touch softly, massage, or drum over the area of interest and set my intentions to healing this area. I find that I pull out drumming or tapping skills over areas that I feel need breaking up. That might be energetically or physically. I love to create a flow of movement to interfere with the current patterns that might be set there. You can drum down your entire body if you need a reset of energy or drum strictly on the area that is in pain. For you to release your own muscle aches and issues, the key is all about awareness and intention. It really does come down to that, no matter the avenue you choose for release and reset.

Drumming

Drumming with your cupped hands along your body, especially on your back or over the chest and lung area, can help you to let go of negative energies hanging out in your body. Drum over the areas that might feel tight or heavy. Drum over it to break up the energetic area, and breathe deeply into this space if possible to help the broken-up pieces leave the body. Let the energy flow out of you through the hands, feet, mouth, top of the head, and ears. Allow the drumming to continue into other parts of the body until you have drummed over all areas that you can reach on your own. While you drum, pair this with intention and words. Talk to your body. Feel whatever is under your hands and help it release with the movement of the drumming hands. Let the vibration break it up and push it out.

Writing

Writing things down can be so cathartic. Write your story. Write your intentions. Write your goals. Write your angers. If you write things you want to release, then be sure to release the paper by burying it or burning it. If you are writing to ease your mind, free your spirit, or honor your creative joys, save your writing and continue adding to it. Keep a journal. Don't judge yourself when you write in your journal. Don't edit. Just be raw and honest. It's yours and no one else needs to see it. Vomit the information and don't look back. Keep turning the pages and move forward in your life, in your growth, and in your writing.

Rituals

There are many things that each individual practices that, overtime, become a ritual. Some people do rituals to their homes for protection. Some of these include pouring salt around the entire home's perimeter.

You can also place a bowl of sea salt or salt water below the bed where you sleep. At night when you lie down, allow all of the negative energy that you experienced or witnessed to fall off your body from the back side down into the bowl beneath the bed. Allow the salt to purify the energy and take it away from you. Let every thought simply drop down into it. Let it go and do not pick it back up in the morning.

A ritual can include being outside at night and burning sage, other herbs, or a paper that you have written the thing you intend to release. I personally love to take out paper and write my intentions on them and then burn them along with frankincense (brings in divine energy and earth energy), amber (releases serious negative energy), myrrh (grounding and bringing in divine energy), sage (cleansing/protecting), or black salt (protection).

Honestly, your ritual might be weekly wine night with friends. Not all rituals have to be set in the deepest nights or under the moon or anything like that. It is something sacred to you to help you heal. However you go about doing that, keep it healthy, stay focused, and honor your intentions for whatever you are taking part in.

To Center—Stretching with Intention

Knowing that my muscles hurt physically and knowing the emotional component of my soreness helps me to be able to work through my own muscles with intention and movement. Taking my neck through a series of stretches where I hold each end of the stretch and then breathe into the space of tension. Hold the spots that ache and then as you exhale, allow the emotions and the physical tensions to leave either through the soles of your feet or out the palms of your hands. I might hold my head with one hand and extend the other arm out with my palm facing up. I allow the energy to leave through my open palm. Energy leaves through the hands, the feet, the ears, the mouth, the bowels, the urine, the nose, and through the top of the head. Anything that can move physically out of your body, so too moves the energy. Much of this can be done simply with the intention behind knowing you are willing to release and move it out. Stretching is something that will come up much more in part 2.

Invocation

When engaging in energy practice, it is important to be very clear with your intentions. Creating a sacred space is of the utmost importance. Other affirmations you may want to consider are:

- I ask the white light to surround me now.
- I am safe, protected, and loved.
- I am in a safe, healing space and all actions lead to my greatest good and highest joys.
- Peace and healing to all involved.

Part II
Emotional Component for Each Muscle Group

❧

Chapter 4

The Back

Your Storehouse for Betrayal,
Protection, and Support

Have you ever felt "stabbed in the back"? There is a reason it is dubbed with this title. The back muscles are a storehouse for stress, grief, sorrow, fear, and, most of all, betrayal. There are ways to finally remove those old wounds and move forward without all of that pain that is so often kept hidden underneath the shoulder blades (especially the right one). This chapter outlines the back muscles and offers ways to find relief from muscle stiffness, pain, and discomfort once and for all.

Back pain is a common complaint among adults, and it's no wonder—the back is a mighty array of muscles that house some of our most negative and unpleasant emotions, from our memories of past betrayals to the sorrow of present grief. There are superficial muscles and deep muscles running all along and throughout the back, and the emotions that hide beneath these massive muscles can cause severe tension and stiffness if not treated and released.

The back represents our structure of support. Our spine along with the back muscles support us in every aspect of our lives, so it's important to keep your back healthy and free of physical and emotional tension. There are many muscles on the back, but it's the muscles that hold the most emotionally charged information that interest us here, so we will focus primarily on these most common and most often problematic trouble spots: the trapezius, the muscles of the scapula, the paraspinals, and the muscles of the lower back.

The Trapezius, aka the Traps

When we think of this muscle, we think of the tops of our shoulders, but the trapezius actually covers a much larger area. Starting from the top of the neck, this muscle comes out to the very ends of each shoulder and makes its way down in a V form all the way to the twelfth rib. It's a humongous muscle, and it's also the back's most superficial muscle—meaning that it lies on top of other muscles that run underneath at different directions. This is the muscle that houses our stress and tension.

Every person—and I do mean literally every person—that goes in for a massage complains of the stress they keep in the shoulder areas of the trapezius. There are two major reasons for this muscle being such a culprit of pain. At the physical level, because we sit upright without using proper posture at all times, this muscle begins to cramp up. Sitting in a stiff chair all day staring at a computer screen does take its toll! The second main culprit of pain in the trapezius is emotional. If you are someone who absolutely must be in charge, you might find it challenging to release stress and relax. This pent-up tension can lead to major pain in the trapezius. Incidentally, moms are notorious for having issues in this muscle!

Many times when we refer to feeling the weight of the world on your shoulders, we are really focusing on the trapezius group. Emotionally, it implies that things have piled onto us. Often when people carry that stress and overwhelmed feelings in this area, it is unintentionally brought on themselves. People with the most issues in this area tend to be type A personality… perfectionist, controlling, or untrusting. Maybe you don't let go of the reins and believe that only you are capable of doing things the way you want them to be done. This is a big deal because it is a self-perpetuated issue. While it is entirely possible that it is totally physical and you do carry your purse only on one arm all the time and your purse is ridiculously heavy, it is important to examine your tendencies and own them where they need to be held. When people complain about shoulder pain, they often point to the trapezius muscle—not the deltoids. Or they refer to tightness in their neck and shoulders. This location again is actually the top of the traps, which they often blanket term as the shoulders.

The movement for traps are elevation and depression and this holds true deeply into the muscles. The action of the trapezius muscle is elevation—lifting the shoulders upward. When this muscle is activated, it tightens and lifts upward. When the muscle is inactive, however, it should be relaxed and lowered—not tense and hunched up. Ask yourself then if your shoulders and traps happen to be stuck in the active position.

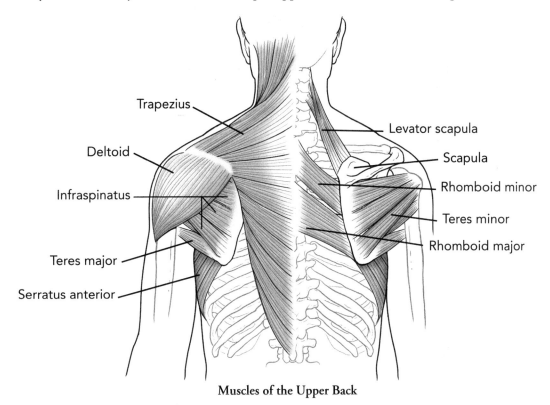

Muscles of the Upper Back

If you are doing a task, the shoulders should be squared to whatever you are facing. There should be room between your chin and your shoulders—perhaps much more room than you are used to having. Although the trapezius muscle can hold amazing amounts of tension, releasing the pain in this area is actually pretty easy.

❀ THE TRAPEZIUS SELF-RELEASE EXERCISE

The secret to helping yourself access and release your muscles is in the knowledge of what the muscle actually does. Knowing that the trapezius muscles' action is elevation, we can go the opposite route to help it let go and move passively instead. There is a simple trick to accessing your traps and helping them to release on your own.

Make a fist and tighten up your whole arm. Push your fist straight down against a hard, flat surface. If you are standing near a desk, place the flat part of your knuckle on the flat part of your desk and push down. At the same time, slowly lean your head to the opposite side. If you are pushing down with your right hand, for example, stretch your neck so that the left ear goes toward your left shoulder. To increase the effectiveness of this stretch even more, open your mouth comfortably until you feel the stretch go all the way down the neck with a bit of heat.

This exercise will quickly release a lot of the pain and tension that builds up in the shoulder and neck areas of the trapezius. Be mindful when you do this exercise to turn off the traps. Talk to the muscles. Explain to them that although they are tight from all the pressure you feel you are under, they no longer need to carry so much weight inside them. Give them permission to let it go. By saying this either out loud or in your mind to your muscles while doing this stretch you are not only talking to the muscles but you are talking to your mind. You are creating an affirmation with this intention and it helps the whole circle unlock.

This stretch can get the muscles back to their intended range of motion. However, what's really going on is that you also must address the emotional component of what's sitting deep within your traps. You have to learn how to let go of the reins a bit and realize that teamwork needs to become your friend. You may be the best at what you do, but there are many ways to do things and accomplish tasks. As the saying goes: You can tell me what to do or you can tell me how to do it…but you cannot tell me both.

I learned an incredibly valuable lesson when I lived at the yoga ashram while studying. Each day we did something referred to as Karma Yoga. We were assigned certain tasks to do (mine was to clean the bathrooms) to help burn off some of our individual karma. They explained it as "You do this work for God." Therefore, no person should be part of your assignment. The part that was so powerful to me was that no one was allowed to criticize nor praise anyone's work. It was hard not to walk in and say "Wow this looks so good!" or "Hey, you missed a spot!" but it was liberating to let each person do their work and you be no part of it.

You may want to introduce that thought into your psyche. Let go a little bit. We don't always have to attach ourselves to someone else's way of doing something. If it's not super important, delegate it out to someone else. Also, maybe consider trusting other people to do things too. Become better at seeing that your way is not the only way to get something done well. The other thing is, be okay if someone does not do things to your standards. Especially if who you are dealing with are children. Let them do their best and do not go back over and fix it. Celebrate anyone's victories and efforts the best you can. This can become a very powerful lesson. Notice that if you apply it, it will lighten your physical load as well.

Affirmations

When you engage in the self-release exercise, you are targeting the specific muscle group. Adding in the affirmation at the same time connects the body with the mind and strengthens your intentions for the highest outcome. For every affirmation, choose one or more statements that best fits where you are currently or create your own. Repeat the statement throughout the day.

- I no longer need to carry the weight of the world on my shoulders.
- I give what I have when I can with no expectations placed upon myself to give more than this.
- I give all I am able without attachment.
- I am doing the best I can with what I have where I am and so is everybody else.

The Scapula

The scapula, aka the shoulder blades, is not a muscle, but a bone. Attached to it however are eighteen highly used muscles—no wonder you hurt there all the time! What has been referred to in anatomy class as "count scapula," the scapula is an impressive bone, and the muscles that attach to it spread from the front to the back to the sides of the body. As a clinical massage therapist, the number one complaint I hear about in this area is a never-ending tension that hides right underneath the scapula toward the middle of the back.

The scapula houses a very intricate set of muscles, and signs of overuse are often present. Key muscles to pay attention to are the rhomboids that attach to the medial borders of the scapula. These muscles can cause immense tension in people. There is also an area that sits at the very top of that side of the bone as well. At the tip-top of the medial side of the scapula above the rhomboids sits the insertion of a muscle called the levator scapula. This muscle, in my opinion, is a major muscle of note and a real powerhouse of tightness and pain. I relate it to the Great Wall—it's a massive muscle (not in size but in the physical tension that is ever-present) that essentially separates the top traps from the rhomboid. This means it can easily hold the emotional tension of the traps, neck, and shoulders, and just as intensely absorb the emotions of the rhomboid and scapula area of betrayal.

The muscle itself originates at the base of the skull, runs down the neck, and inserts into that top inside corner of the scapula. If you are a therapist, getting your finger right inside the top end of that bone to treat that area can help so much (as well as treating the sternocleidomastoid on the front side to help release the levator scapula).

The neck and the back obviously go hand in hand and releasing one will help unlock the other. However, that physical discomfort is only half of the story. If it's only the physical pain and tension that needs treatment, then why is it that you can go to massage therapists, physical therapists, acupuncturists, chiropractors, and more for relief and nothing seems to change the fact that in only a few days time, the same familiar aches and pains return? This is where the emotions come in—and entirely too many people miss this component because they simply don't know it exists. When we treat the emotional causes as well as the physical symptoms of pain, what we can find is lasting relief—whether it's in the rhomboids, the trapezius, the biceps, the calves, or any other muscle in the body.

The rhomboids and levator scapula are huge culprits for carrying pain and stiffness, both for physical reasons and emotional. These muscles, which lie beneath the trapezius group, are responsible for elevation and to pull toward the midline (levator scapula), pulling the arms back to squeeze your shoulder blades together (rhomboid minor and major), as all are downward rotators.

The muscles of the scapula hold the energetic effects of emotional betrayal, and all that pent-up sadness and suspicion can exacerbate pain in this already overworked area. Have you ever been stabbed in the back? It doesn't have to be something that happened last week—it could be as far back as when you were a teenager and your girlfriend or boyfriend cheated on you, or even further in the past when your parents decided to split without giving you a say in it. Whatever it was that made you feel betrayed, it happened behind your back. Now where in the body do you suppose this heartache is stored? Behind your back, of course—the upper middle part of your back behind your heart. This muscle holds so much emotional energy from past pains, anger, hurt, shame, embarrassment, and, most of all, betrayal. These stored emotions are so much more powerful than you can imagine … until you let them go, and you're hit with the full magnitude of what you were carrying around for so long. Don't forget that this is also your full heart space. So not only is it stored in your back, but it lingers deeply into your heart space. Talking about the emotional pains as the physical pains are being released is extremely helpful in looping it together with your mind effectively.

On a deeper note, I find that pain in the muscles of the right side scapula (where most people hurt worse) indicates a solid betrayal that you did not expect or have a hand in—one that you are, on some level, still angry about. Pain around the left side scapula, however, is a more subtle pain. It may still hurt physically as much as the other side, but it indicates a somewhat different situation. The right side of the body is the giving side, so pain in the muscles of your right scapula could indicate that you are still on some very slight level giving power to the emotional pain of betrayal that is stored in this area of the body. Pain in the muscles of the scapula on the left side of the body, however, could indicate that you have absolutely no idea that you are still harboring the emotional pain that lies at the heart of the situation, and this blissful ignorance makes both the emotional and the physical aspects of the pain much more difficult to pinpoint and treat. You are receiving this pain but not actively involved with it. It requires a more subtle and delicate approach to rid the left side shoulder blade of emotional traumas, and if you are experiencing such pain, you'll need to dig deep with total honesty to discover the true emotional source of the disturbance.

We tend to forgive to the best of our abilities, but in most cases, we never forget. Even if we don't think about it anymore, betrayal is not something that leaves us. Feeling stabbed in the back by friends, lovers, or parents leaves a lasting impression, and we can find it among those shoulder blade muscles exactly where you felt the proverbial knife enter in—right behind the heart. To release your body down to its core, down to the muscles, the last holders of pain, will change your life.

❀ CONNECTING WITH YOUR INNER CHILD
SELF-RELEASE EXERCISE

To get down deep, try this mind practice. There is an old trick to getting answers from your inner child. As I stated, the right and left sides are different with regard to giving and receiving. It goes deeper than this though. Pull out a sheet of paper and write down the questions you are trying to figure out. Write down every question you can think of that might help you pinpoint the pains hidden deeply within. Once you've written all of your questions, change hands. Answer the questions with your nondominant hand. This activates a part of your brain that is your child brain. It does not have the secure gates around the walls of thought. It will surprise you what you write down. Do not give it thought; just let yourself answer the questions with that hand. Once you have some new and deeper information, you can better help yourself let go of old pains that have kept you feeling betrayed and pained. When you look at your answers, try not to judge them. Only learn from them.

Affirmations

When you engage in the self-release exercise, you are targeting the specific muscle group. Adding in the affirmation at the same time connects the body with the mind and strengthens your intentions for the highest outcome. For every affirmation, choose one or more statement that best fits where you are currently or create your own. Repeat the statement throughout the day.

- I release shames and angers from the past.
- I am free to move on without carrying any old knife wounds. The scars may remain, but there is no more pain within them.
- I have removed the knife from my back, and I am free to move into the greatest joys of life with no need to ever look back.
- I can now express my love freely.
- I am love. I give love. I am open to receive love.

The Paraspinals

This is a muscle group that runs parallel with the spine from the lumbar (lower back) to the cervical (neck). There are many muscles that make up the paraspinals and many insertions of each muscle. Some run the entire length of the spine, while others insert at various places along the way.

When people feel that meaty muscle that parallels the spine, they only think of the erectors, but it is all of those muscles that are involved in this long band of muscles. They support your every move.

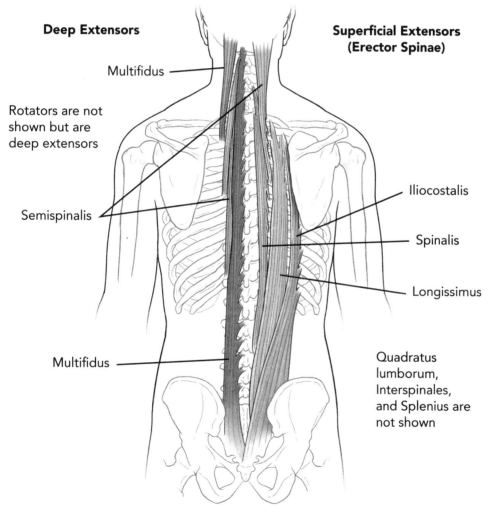

Deep Extensors

Multifidus

Rotators are not shown but are deep extensors

Semispinalis

Multifidus

Superficial Extensors (Erector Spinae)

Iliocostalis

Spinalis

Longissimus

Quadratus lumborum, Interspinales, and Splenius are not shown

The Paraspinals

The paraspinal muscles are your support group. They keep you standing tall and help you to keep going. When we feel weak or in doubt of our path, these muscles may tense up and react to our mental thoughts. These muscles remind you to stand tall, lift your chin up, and keep moving forward. These muscles also protect your kidneys and adrenal glands (the organ storehouse for fear and anxiety). We must be flexible and give our all to everything we put our minds and hearts into. This muscle group will support your movement in your body and in your mind. If you are being treated by a therapist, cross fiber friction is a wonderful tool to use to treat the paraspinals and erectors.

Treating these muscles provides a level of comfort for the body and mind that is hard to describe. It can provide feelings of safety and a deep relief when treated by someone who really knows how to treat these muscles with both the disruption and gentleness that they crave. While I offer in this book self-care techniques and stretches, I also recommend finding a wonderful clinical body worker near you to address areas such as these. They can bring your body so much release that is simply beyond something you can get to and treat manually on your own.

⌘ The Cat/Cow Self-Release Exercise

To open up the full spine and all of the muscles in the back is a very simple cat/cow stretch. On all fours, make sure your hands are directly under your shoulders and flat to the floor. The knees should be directly under the hips. Exhale and look at your belly as you round your back. Inhale and lift the chin up as you open the full chest up and open. Each exhale, look down as your back rounds, and each inhale, lift the chest up as the chin looks up toward the ceiling. On the exhale, feel the full back lift up toward the heavens as it exposes each vertebrae, allowing them to stretch and gain space between each one. When you inhale and lift the chest, feel the love energy enter directly into your heart space. When you exhale, try to blow the energy into your stomach and heart space. Take the love in through your heart on the inhale, give the love back to your heart on the exhale. As you round the back, tuck the chin tightly in and breathe out all the stagnant chi that has been lying dormant.

Cat Pose

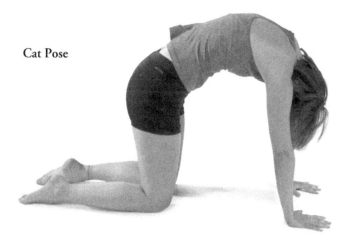

Cow Pose

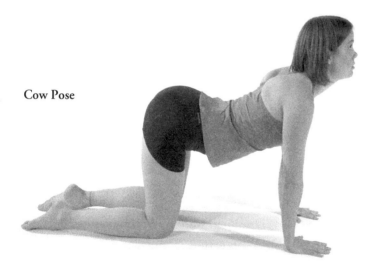

Affirmations

When you engage in the self-release exercise, you are targeting the specific muscle group. Adding in the affirmation at the same time connects the body with the mind and strengthens your intentions for the highest outcome. For every affirmation, choose one or more statement that best fits where you are currently or create your own. Repeat the statement throughout the day.

- I am strong and I am supple.
- I move forward in my life with grace and dignity.
- I am flexible, willing, and able.
- I move freely with ease.
- I trust the process.
- I am in alignment with Divine guidance.

The Muscles of the Lower Back

Lower back pain causes issues for so many of us! From the physical discomfort to the limitations in flexibility and mobility, lower back pain is serious business. Physically, there are many explanations for it, and, although the emotional causes are equally important to examine, it's absolutely vital to understand the physical mechanics of what's going on with your body as well. The meat of muscle that goes from the bottom of the twelfth rib to the top of the low back bones in the pelvic girdle are known as the quadratus lumborum (QL). These muscles physically govern upright movement and side-to-side motion (meaning leaning to the side). The opposite muscle group on the front side are your abdominals and your oblique abdominals. More so, however, lies the psoas as the counter to the low back muscles. The psoas is serious business, both physically and emotionally.

When we understand what's going on with our bodies both emotionally and physically, we're able to identify problematic behaviors and change habits that might otherwise exacerbate the pain. For example, one of the most common causes of back pain is an excessive curvature of the spine. The spine is naturally curved, but scoliosis (a sideways curve of the spine), lordosis (excessive inward curve of the spine or sway back), and kyphosis (an abnormally convex curvature of the spine) are issues that deal with a more severe or off-center curvature of the spine.

I myself have a sway back. When I was a gymnast, I had a stress fracture in my lower back. These two problems together have resulted in an enormous amount of pain throughout the years. However, as my knowledge about the body grew, I came to understand the physical components of the pain and was able to find ways to reduce and manage the discomfort. I adjusted my posture and started choosing proper footwear—two simple, very physical solutions that help tremendously. Also if your lower back is weak, you must strengthen your core. Today, I'm aware of the emotional causes of my lower back pain in addition to the physical causes, and I can therefore take a more complete, more holistic approach to my treatment.

When it comes to emotions of the lower back it is twofold. The low back area itself, especially in the sacrum (the triangular shaped bone at the base of the spine), is considered the sacred bone. It can hold a great amount of fear. The sacrum at its worst deals with financial security fears and moving forward in your life. It also deals with loss of people, which gives way to fears of moving forward without that particular person or situation. At its best, this area can shed the fears and help you to become the very strong and capable person that I know you can be. At best in the sacrum and low back area, you can connect into your soul space and tap into your own path toward your greatest opportunities moving forward.

It is important to note that attached to the lumbar area of the spine but from the part that faces the stomach happens to be the origin of the iliopsoas muscle. If you recall at the beginning of the book, my massage teacher had explained that the psoas muscle is one of the most emotional muscles in the body. We will discuss the psoas in its own chapter, but having such a pull to the lower back is an important connection you need to keep in mind and be aware of. If the lower back spasms or seizes up, it is the psoas that we treat to release the back. They are so intimately connected both physically and emotionally that you must consider both when treating the physical aspects of the lower back.

To finally address and try to let go of months or even years of grief isn't usually very pretty, and it's generally accomplished through a combination of awareness and a good, hard cry—in other words, by acknowledging the emotional component of the pain and crying it out. When we cry a wholehearted, gut-wrenching, emotion-releasing cry, often we cannot help but bend over at the waist. The tears feel as if they are produced way down in the feet, working their way with extreme sorrow up the legs, through the back, up into the chest, and finally out of the eyes in a gust of uncontrollable emotion. There is no way to stand up tall and grieve in this way. Bending forward at the waist allows that lower back to open itself up and let go of the emotional pain it harbors, helping the cry be more productive through the release of all that sadness and grief that has been housed within your body.

Many people when truly grieving curl up in a fetal position or lie in child's pose. Part of the reason we do this is to expose that lower back so that it can let go of the built-up emotional pain right along with you. The lower back is an area of deep internal aware-ness, and only through powerful emotional release can the pain be truly healed. This also goes hand in hand with the psoas and its connection to the autonomic nervous system. Curling up in a fetal position elicits the freeze response when faced with fight, flight, or freeze when our bodies become overwhelmed or faced with perceived danger. In facing this level of trauma, the freeze response has been activated.

❀ The Child's Pose Self-Release Exercise

The child's pose is one you can do very easily. Gently sit back on your heels and bring your arms down by your feet or you can keep the hands extended above the head. This exposes the low back, and you can remain in a very easy, sacred space in doing so.

Child's Pose

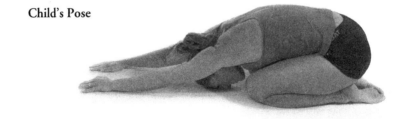

⌘ Additional Low Back Release Exercise

Lying on your back, gently lift one knee deeply into the chest. Wrap both of your arms around that bent knee. Change legs and bend the other knee into the chest and straighten the other leg. Hold each bent leg into the chest for a minimum of five deep breaths. Then bring both knees into the chest and wrap your arms so tightly around the knees so that the knees and ankles touch together and you reach to grab around each elbow of the arms. Keep your head on the ground and your chin slightly tucked in. Gently roll side to side to truly acknowledge your lower back. Lift your head and kiss the knee. Hold this pose for three deep breaths or more before lowering the head back down. Change legs and repeat.

Knee into Chest

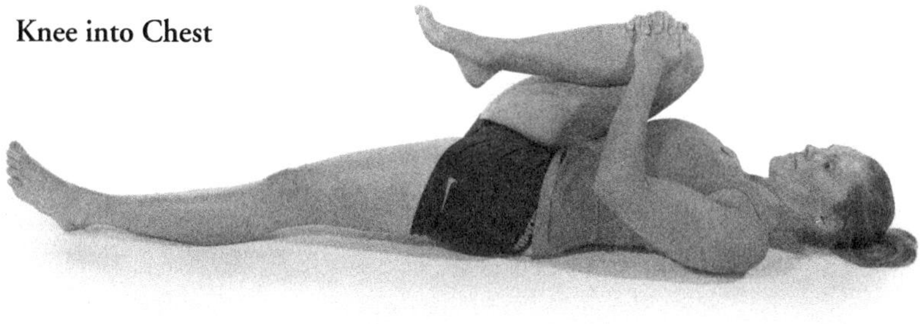

Kissing the Knee

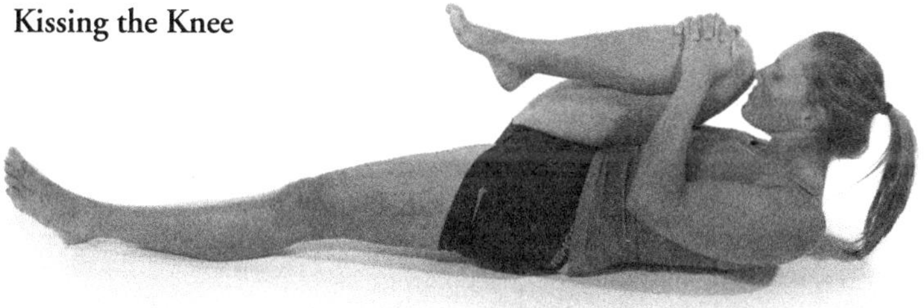

Affirmations

When you engage in the self-release exercise, you are targeting the specific muscle group. Adding in the affirmation at the same time connects the body with the mind and strengthens your intentions for the highest outcome. For every affirmation, choose one or more statement that best fits where you are currently or create your own. Repeat the statement throughout the day.

- I am able to move forward with my life without fear of financial worry.
- The Universe will provide for me, and I will do my part in my own success.
- I take responsibility for my life and my choices with grace and gratitude.
- I have love in my heart and joy in my body as I embrace change and fluid motion of forward movement.
- I am open and available to heal from the deepest depths of my being *now.*

Suggested Stones for the Back

Black tourmaline: A protection stone thought to create a force field of energy around the entire body for protection.

Carnelian: Helps to strengthen the back. It is associated with lower back pains and helping to strengthen the area on an energetic level.

Jet: Helps dispel fears and negative patterns as well as awaken the kundalini energy in the spine.

Rose quartz: Worn in necklace form to protect the heart chakra/upper middle back and to send loving energy to the corresponding area in the back for clearing and healing.

Suggested Essential Oils for the Back

Try **jasmine, frankincense, ylang ylang, lavender, rose,** or **sandalwood** for the lower back and the corresponding chakras (first and second).

For upper chakra (third through fifth) neck issues, suggested oils are **lavender** or **chamomile** for evening or **peppermint** for daytime. Place a couple drops on the back of the neck or add to carrier oils and massage into the neck. Remember the mint family is not to be put directly onto the skin without dilution.

✵ Meditation for Clearing, Releasing, and Protecting the Entire Back

The back is the part of your energetic body that does not have the level of armor that you do in the front. Therefore, energy work to the back can heal the heart center easier than if you had your hands placed from the front. The back is an open and vital entryway to the chakras to clear and cleanse.

For this meditation, I ask that you lie down in child's pose, exposing your back by kneeling and then sitting your bottom on your heels, placing your forehead down on the ground, and allowing your arms to lay by your sides or extended above your head. Feel the back in this position allowing it to be totally rounded, open, and exposed. Close your eyes and allow your breathing to bring energy into the back with each breath in, on the exhale release any tension, sadness, shame, and/or fears. Imagine that between the shoulder blades opens up a door energetically, like shutters opening your heart area, as well as allowing the muscles and emotions along the spine to open up completely. Imagine an incredible green color emanating from deep within and exposing itself up and out through these open doors that your back has created.

In your mind's eye, see an emerald green circle of energy coming up and out of your middle back, a giant ball of green blobby energy pulling from every vertebrae, every part of your entire back up and down. Imagine that this energy is taking with it any wounds, or even knives, still left in that space. Envision these unwanted pains rising up and out as the green circle of energy grows larger. See yourself playing, massaging, or ringing out the old, unwanted energy the way you would wring out a wet washcloth. Watch the green circle as things drop out of this energy blob that no longer serves any positive purpose in your body. Anything that drops off the blob does not fall back into your body but rather is dropped and then evaporates into the ether before it ever gets back to you. Keep kneading and shaping this blobby circle until it becomes clear green or bright emerald green, depending on your energy and perception.

Bring back the energy of your original, authentic childlike self who is clearer, softer, kinder. Then place it back inside your own body healed, renewed, and with a new awareness to stay open, clean, and peaceful.

Chapter 5

The Glutes

Your Storehouse for Aggravation and Suppression

The function of the gluteus maximus, medius, and minimus muscles (or glutes) is to stabilize the pelvis. When you lift one foot, the glutes stabilize the spine and keep you upright. Gluteus maximus is a hip extensor, and it is strong and powerful. It allows you to do movements such as jumping and climbing stairs. The gluteus minimus and medius muscles work together as a medial rotator of the thigh and serve as a cushion for the pelvis while in a seated position. They are also abductor muscles that bring the leg out from the center line.

Another muscle of note is the piriformis muscle. The piriformis is a major lateral rotator of the hip. It is antagonistic to the glute medius and minimus, which serve as a medial rotator and abductor of the thigh. This muscle starts in the sacrum (I'm simplifying the origin and insertion details of this muscle down to the very basics) and inserts on the greater trochanter (that bone you can feel on the side of your thigh). I think of this muscle as being shaped like a slice of pizza. The piriformis muscle has the sciatic nerve running beneath it, and boy does this muscle cause some issues! When the piriformis muscle gets too tight, it can compress the sciatic nerve, which can lead to major pain and limited motion. If you are having physical issues in this area, consider going to a licensed massage therapist who can really get in there deep to release the tension.

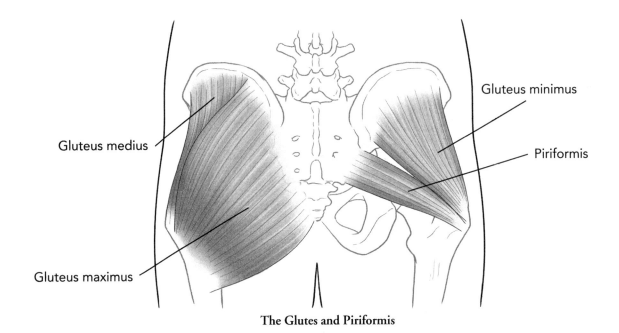

Gluteus minimus

Gluteus medius

Piriformis

Gluteus maximus

The Glutes and Piriformis

Emotionally, the glutes are associated with aggravation and suppression. Can you recall all of those times that something made you really angry but it just wasn't worth actually bringing up? Or maybe you were in a place where that angry situation occurred and you absolutely could not express your dismay? So you sit on it for a bit. Sometimes you sit on it and do nothing with it. Sometimes you sit on it and chew it up and spit it out and chew it up some more in your head and you still deem it absolutely not worth having the conversation about. Hopefully if you do give a situation that much thought, you do end up discussing it and trying to heal it. Even still, if you've been sitting on it for a while, the emotional pain has had time to make its way in and bury deep into this area. Those emotions that we sat on…we literally did sit on it! They are now stored as aggravation and suppression in your glutes.

In order to free those emotions, it takes acknowledging that this is what is actually going on. It's one thing to have the muscles themselves released, and it's another thing entirely when you release not only the muscles but also the pent-up emotions that lurk within those muscles. When you heal the emotional as well as the physical, that's when the tension doesn't come back as easily. This allows you to start fresh and sit on brand-new emotions! Hopefully experiencing a new lightness in your bum will make you more aware of the way that you digest outside information and manage it.

In the introduction, I discussed my client whom I had worked on for quite a while and the suppression she felt in her gluteus shortly after her ex-husband had passed away. "What made you think about that now?" I asked. "I've worked on you for almost forty-five minutes now; what made you think of this now while I'm working in this particular area?" She shrugged and said, "I don't know. It just came to me." I would have had no way of knowing that this situation was happening in her life. She had no way of knowing that this is where her pent-up anger was hiding out. For her, it doesn't matter where that pent-up anger is hanging out, it only matters that I can escort it out. After she told me of this situation, the muscles let up. We must acknowledge our feelings and experiences and then allow any unwanted emotional tension to leave the body.

Inhale and think about what it is that is annoying you, then exhale with a mighty breath and let those feelings leave. Do this repeatedly. Another way to help this along is to write down your feelings whenever you feel frustrated or angry, but don't plan to talk about it out loud. Write it down and tear it up or burn it or keep it for another time, or to add-on to. The most important piece of this is acknowledging the emotions so you can let them go.

When I'm doing body work on a client and I know it's emotional, I let the person know that the feelings they are experiencing as they come up are valid and not random. When the muscles start firing and shaking, and they start fidgeting and trying to get more comfortable, I know it's emotional. That is one of the first signs that the emotions have been trapped and that they are slowly and angrily trying to escape the muscle they have been held captive under.

We become attached to our emotions and sometimes we just don't want to let it out. The client will start to fidget—they don't realize it, but their body is trying to find a new place where that emotion can safely hide out. It's as if they're trying to stuff that emotion into another drawer in the body. Remember back in the beginning of the book when I described the Apothecary Method? The person, when faced with discomfort, will try to move the emotional sensation (as well as physical pain) into another part of the body.

You must watch their body for subtle movements in order to help them clean house. This can be done through energy work, intention, breathing, acknowledging, manual therapies, crying, coughing, and other releasing techniques. It is also important to check in with your client to be sure you are not going too deep with your pressure and lighten when needed. (See chapter 4 for more information.)

⌘ The Foam Roller Self-Release Exercise

If you have a foam roller or even a tennis ball, use it to find the spots on your glutes that are the most sensitive. Place the roller or the ball under that area and gently move back and forth over it or just sit on that spot until it lightens up. *Search and treat* is the motto for this work. Move over the muscles at an angle, mostly targeting gluteus minimus and medius. Do this with intention. Speak to your muscles, allowing them to release those pent-up angers and resentments. In this space, it's not the time to go softly along. The glutes will open the door to that low back stuff as well, so keep moving with the ball or roller. Get that full body release. On your exhales, open your mouth wide and either yell or do a very loud sigh. You have to play an active role in this.

One of the most effective and easiest ways to release the emotion stored in the glutes is to go for a nice loud YELL. Yell it out! Get it out of your body and out of those angry muscles. Start with meeting the emotion with like emotions. Give it the strength and stamina to be let out. Think of a lion's roar. Get aggressive in here. Be bold; talk louder than usual in this space when working to release from this area. This is not the time for sweet talking and comforting the emotions out like in some of the other parts of the body. This area has been suppressed long enough and these emotions deserve to be given a voice. Allow your voice to resonate with power and dominance.

Affirmations

When you engage in the self-release exercise, you are targeting the specific muscle group. Adding in the affirmation at the same time connects the body with the mind and strengthens your intentions for the highest outcome. For every affirmation, choose one or more statement that best fits where you are currently or create your own. Repeat the statement throughout the day.

- I am free to let go of all the times I did not honor my feelings and sat them out.
- I embrace a new way of communicating, where I speak my truth freely and kindly so that things do not fester within my being.
- I am free to move into a higher space of consciousness.
- Angers and frustrations no longer have a place to be planted within me.
- I release the frustrations and walk away with ease and peace.

Suggested Stones for the Glutes

Amazonite: A stone of communication, integrity, hope, and trust. It is said to stimulate the throat chakra, and it's associated with strong, honest communication. This is a powerful stone to have nearby when doing this release work. Whatever stones you choose, don't choose obsidian stones. They magnify your emotions, so keep these stones away for now.

Blue kyanite: Can help dispel feelings of anger and frustration. When using kyanite, do not share this stone. If you do, clean it thoroughly. This balances and aligns the chakras and helps the anger move out smoothly.

Carnelian: Helps to protect you and empower you, allowing you to carry through emotions like anger. It is an excellent stone for the back side of the body.

Hematite: A powerful grounding stone. When you are flighty, angry, or generally out of balance, use this stone on your ankles, at your feet, and around your wrists. Be powerful in your body.

Suggested Essential Oils for the Glutes

All oils are suggested to be used through a diffuser and not directly on your skin unless you already know how to mix it with a carrier oil and you're positive that the oil is nontoxic and safe to use on the skin.

Bergamot: Can calm and help alleviate worry and distrust. *Do not use bergamot directly on the skin.

Frankincense: Can help you stand in line with your own power, especially when you are angry. This oil will help ground you and empower you and carry you through the angry emotions.

Lavender: This is always your safe oil for calming down.

Myrrh: Uplifts the spirit and helps dispel anger.

Orange: Calms, uplifts, inspires a brighter attitude, and helps release stress and worry.

Ylang Ylang: Is a sweet, flowery scent that calms the nerves and soothes the soul.

⌘ Meditation for Clearing, Releasing, and Protecting the Glutes

Those glutes have been holding on to those feelings for a very long time. Take your time with this exercise. The hope is that by the end you either come up energized and renewed or you go to the best release of all and cry it out. No judgment here, it's all about you being able to search and destroy the anger and aggravation you've allowed to be within you for so long.

First you have to get physical so that the muscles in the glutes know you are talking directly to them. Make fists with your hands and beat like a drum beat all over your bottom. Feel the muscles move in response to your fists doing a drum beat over them. Shake it up in there and get the muscles and emotions moving. Maybe go to YouTube and play the old 1980s' song "The Warrior" by Patty Smyth for a little extra power and pleasure while you give all of your attention into this space. If that song doesn't work for you, put in another song that is strong and powerful. Dance if you feel led to. Get your body moving as you continue to drum on that area with your clenched fists. Be physical before you enter a deeper, calmer space.

After a few minutes or one full song of movement, sit down on those muscles and let them tell you their secrets. Sit at your computer or at a desk with a pad of paper and a pencil. Write anything that comes into your mind as the area releases the tension and vibration. The muscles do speak; this is the time to listen. You have gone in there and shaken it up, given them your undivided attention. Now it's time for you to listen to them. Write anything, draw anything, whatever comes into your mind, put it down on paper. This is a way to develop a greater communication with your body. From here, work to create something that is just yours that helps you better listen to what the muscles are trying to tell you.

Chapter 6

The Legs
Your Storehouse for
Moving Forward or Staying Stuck

In this chapter, we will discuss both the muscles of the legs, as well as their emotional counterparts. The legs make up the largest muscle group. This is the area of our body that generates the most power physically. When it comes to the legs, it's all about moving forward or staying stuck. So many of us always feel like we are trying to catch up to our lives. There are so many things to do and not enough time to do them. We are not investing ourselves in the present moments. There is no time to just stop, breathe, and think *This is exactly where I want to be. I am going to take it in and enjoy this very moment.* This occurs in the legs. Always on the run, trying to get to the next thing on our lists. Or if we feel depleted by our life, we want to collapse and stop. That also happens within the legs. When it comes to the legs as a whole, the muscles are what move us and drive us. It is our joints that act up when we feel stuck in the muck. If we feel stuck in quicksand, not knowing which next step to take, it shows up in the knees the most and the ankles and the hips as well.

Our legs take us where we want and need to go, literally moving us forward in the world as we also move forward in life. While it would be great to say that we're always indeed moving forward, sometimes we find ourselves feeling like we're stuck in quicksand, going nowhere or facing setback after setback. Even when we desire so strongly to move forward, we are sometimes resistant to change and our hesitancy in embracing the new prevents us from taking steps toward a better future. When you are having trouble moving to the next phase in life, feeling stuck in the past or mired in the muck of a current struggle, the emotional burdens that keep you weighted down and immobile can manifest as pain and discomfort in the legs. The muscles on the front side of the legs tend to hold the emotional stress associated with issues that lie ahead of you in your future, while the muscles on the backsides of the legs can harbor the pains of traumas that happened in your past. The backside muscles are a little bit more protective and deal with things that are coming up from behind, such as the fear of getting blindsided.

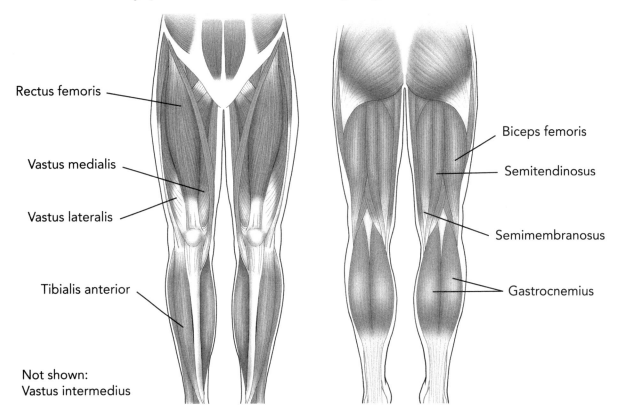

Rectus femoris

Vastus medialis

Vastus lateralis

Tibialis anterior

Not shown:
Vastus intermedius

Biceps femoris

Semitendinosus

Semimembranosus

Gastrocnemius

Overview of the Full Legs—Front and Back

Take a look at the diagram of the legs and you'll see just how many muscles it takes working together in unison to move your body even one step forward. Our emotional bodies are similar. It can be challenging to takes steps toward a better future when we are still feeling the pain of the past or experiencing the fear of what lies ahead. And let's be honest…who's to say it is a better future, anyway? We don't know what lies ahead and that can be really scary. There are a million times where getting to that better place involves some really messy meantime moments.

By gaining a greater awareness of each of your many leg muscles as well as the emotional triggers that might be associated with these muscles, you'll begin to find new ways to release both the physical and emotional pain that has been holding you back. When our legs are feeling good and we're not feeling anchored by the past or stressed out by the future, it's a whole lot easier to actively move ahead and optimistically embrace the new. The goal to keep yourself from feeling like you're standing in quicksand is to keep moving, even if it's in little tiny steps. Take each step that lights up and shows you the way. You don't have to see the whole staircase, just each next step.

Quadriceps

The quadriceps, or quads, are the muscles on the front of the leg above the knee. There are four of them: rectus femoris, vastus medialis, vastus lateralis, and vastus intermedius. The quads are not just muscles that guide movement forward. They play more of a role of connectors. Issues with the knees, hips, or psoas will often be reflected as pain in the quads.

As a generalization, the legs as a whole do deal with our ability to move forward in our lives, but when it comes to the muscles above the knees and below the waist like the quads, be aware that there may be a little more to the story hiding beneath the surface. It is interesting to note that rectus femoris extends the leg at the knee and flexes the hip. The other three muscles only extend the leg at the knee. This is because rectus femoris crosses two joints—the knee and the hips.

The quads are protector muscles. They can help you jump up or stop fast. They bend down low and power up when you go high. They are solid and massive. They protect you when you feel stuck and don't know which way to go. They propel you forward when a new opportunity comes up. The hips point the way forward and the knees and the ankles line up to make that move happen. But the quads are what move you there.

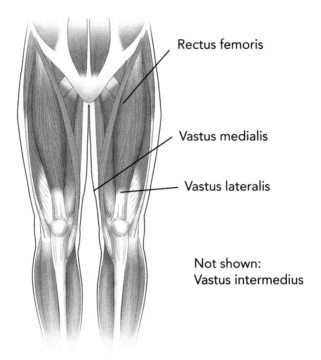

Rectus femoris

Vastus medialis

Vastus lateralis

Not shown:
Vastus intermedius

The Quads

The quads are muscles of trust and power. When you are in alignment with your heart and your head, the quads will take care of you. When you are in chaos, confused, or troubled, the quads will slow you down and become heavy, and you won't be able to feel their power quite the same. You'll have to play the role of the mystery solver and stay open to what your muscles and emotions are telling you to determine exactly what is the real underlying issue in these areas. Think of the quads as a band of horses and you are holding the reins. When you need to giddyyap and get going, you have to pull on the reins and give the command. If you are not in motion, they will lay down and take a rest. These are power muscles and they need to be fed. This lines up with your mind and your ability to make decisions without vacillating back and forth. Be strong in your mind, take charge of your life and your body, and put those quads in motion.

❀ THE QUADS SELF-RELEASE EXERCISE

Perform this stretch gently and as often as is comfortable to help release physical and emotional tension held in the quads. Stand up and hold on to something for balance, gently bring your foot behind you, and hold it in your hand. Hold your right foot in your right hand, then when you're ready, switch, bringing your right foot back down to the floor and bringing your left foot up behind you to hold it in your left hand. Talk to your muscles as you do this stretch and allow them the release both physically and emotionally.

The Quad Stretch

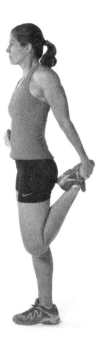

Be open to the emotions and images that are coming to you, and notice how the energy in your quads responds to your thoughts and movements. As you inhale, imagine that you are breathing in light, and as you exhale, visualize the pain and tension releasing from this area, flowing outward and away from your body. These muscles and the emotional memories they hold can become very dense, so be patient with yourself and know that releasing these areas can take some time.

It may take several stretching sessions to even begin to break up that density, but don't overdo it, and continue to be gentle with yourself both physically and emotionally. If you want to bring the hip flexors in with this stretch, all you have to do is add a push-pull move. With the foot in your hand try to pull the foot toward your glutes. At the same time try to push your foot against your hand away from the glutes. This activates the quads and brings in the psoas in a super easy way.

Hamstrings

The semitendinosus, semimembranosus, and biceps femoris are the muscles more commonly known as the hamstrings, and they mainly flex the knee. The hamstrings are not highly emotional muscles. They are emotionally likened to having a body guard with you at all times. They stand strong, they keep you protected, and they are rather stoic. Running right up to the glutes at the sit bone (ischial tuberosity is the point of attachment) and affecting the lower back and all the way down to the calves, the hamstrings are closely linked to tension and tightness in other parts of the legs. Your hips and glutes depend on your hamstrings and vice versa, and something as simple as wearing the wrong sort of shoes can cause the hamstrings to become stiff, painful, and shortened. It's important to give these muscles support as they support so much of the body.

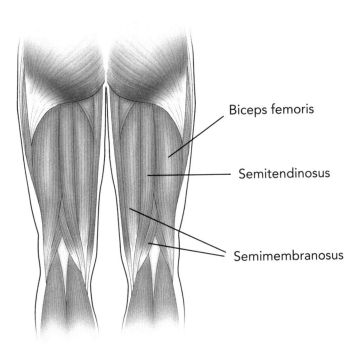

Biceps femoris

Semitendinosus

Semimembranosus

The Hamstrings

⌘ The Hamstrings Self-Release Exercise

As a rule, *contract, relax,* and *stretch* are great tools for any of these muscles in the body—especially for the hamstrings. The legs can get aggressive with you, and they don't like to give up any emotional component that comes with them. *Contract* means to tighten the muscle, then *relax* that muscle to allow you to better *stretch* the muscle.

The Hamstring Stretch—Part 1

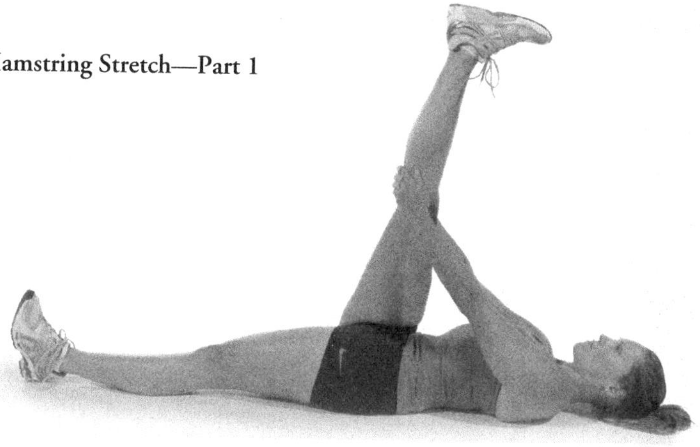

The Hamstring Stretch—Part 2

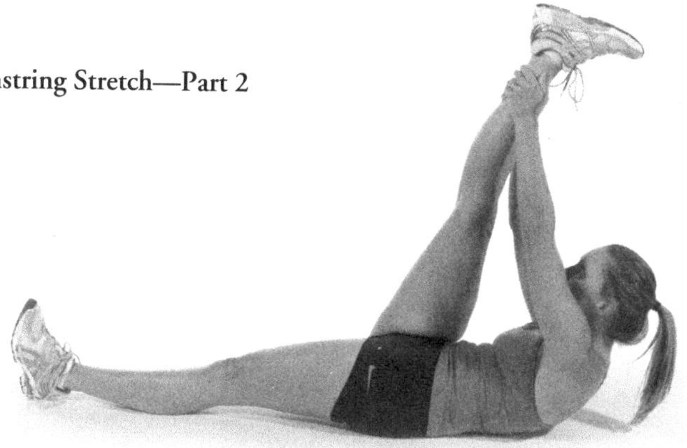

The Hamstring Stretch—Part 3

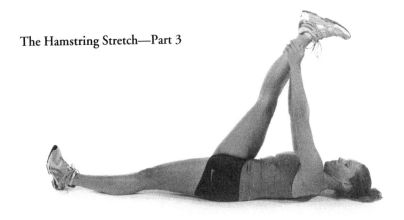

The best self-release stretch for the hamstrings is done lying on your back. Lift one leg up and hold on to it just below or above the knee with both hands. Let the other leg lie straight out on the floor. Keep your head down, inhale, and hold your breath for the contract portion of the stretch. Hold the leg as you tighten the muscle and use your hands as a brace. Your hands are trying to bring the leg toward your head. At the same time, the hamstrings flex and try to push against the hands. Gently relax the leg, continuing to hold it straight up in the air with your hands and exhale.

Now gently try to bring the leg in closer to your body, but do not allow the leg to bend. If your knee bends, bring the leg back to a space where it can remain straight so that the focus is solely on the hamstring group. To increase the stretch, lift your head up and walk your hands up higher toward your foot. Now keep the leg exactly where it is in your hands, lower your head back down, and notice that the stretch increases even more.

Change legs and do this again. With each stretch sequence, focus totally on the hamstrings. These are three muscles that don't like to give it up. Talk to them and thank them for their incredibly solid support in your life. Let them know that they are allowed to take breaks and rest too.

Knees

When thinking of the knee itself, we think of the patella—the bony prominence. But there are so many muscles and tendons that surround the knee that we need to address. It is important to see all of the muscles that surround the knee in both the front and the back of the knee.

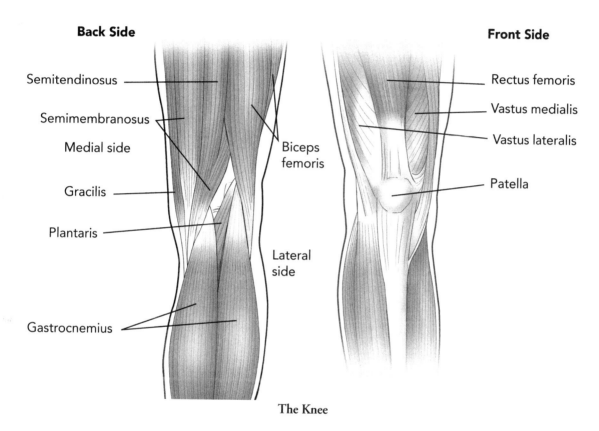

Back Side

Semitendinosus

Semimembranosus

Medial side

Gracilis

Plantaris

Gastrocnemius

Biceps femoris

Lateral side

Front Side

Rectus femoris

Vastus medialis

Vastus lateralis

Patella

The Knee

When it comes to emotional tension that is held in the legs, the knees are where you are likely to feel the most of what is really going on down deep. When we have issues with our knees, we might feel like we're standing in quicksand, like it's very hard to lift your feet and move in any direction. You may feel completely stuck. This might occur when you're facing big changes in your life or whenever things are changing around you and you don't have much of a say in it.

To me the knees are your messengers of how you are experiencing change. If you are resistant, the knees will be the area that begins to hurt, stiffen up, and ache. When people complain of knee issues, I do associate that with a rigidity to life, a resistance to change, or a lack of movement in any direction. It's a standstill. You must be flexible with your knees and your directions, and you must involve your mind in getting back into the groove of life.

❀ THE KNEES SELF-RELEASE EXERCISE

The knee is the largest joint in the body. The energy pattern of the knee is different from the areas of the leg that contain muscles. Therefore, for self-practice, we must energize the knee joint, tendons, and ligaments manually to help the energy flow to this area.

The Knee Stretch

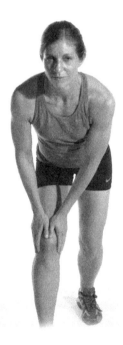

Put one leg in front and keep the body weight to the back leg. Slightly bend the front knee. Cup the hands and place the thumbs over the knee cap as the remainder of the cupped palm covers the entire knee. Be soft in your hands and keep your knee open and soft. Rub up and down over the knee, first gently and

THE LEGS | 103

then speeding up and creating heat over the knee. Feel the knee joints and bones relax into this stimulation of the knee.

Keep your knees comfortable and be patient and mindful. A lot of information can be obtained when you connect to the energy of your knees. Rub your hands up and down over the surface of each knee no less than ten times. The best way is not to keep count and don't stop until there is a great heat and the whole area feels incredibly open and energized. Once you have done the rubbing down of the knee, bring your legs hip-width apart. Bend your knees and keep them bent. Place your hands just above your knees and circle your knees in full circles without straightening back up. Do this ten times in one direction and ten times in the other direction.

Calves: The Muscles of the Gastrocnemius and Soleus

There are two bellies that make up the gastrocnemius—the medial head gastrocnemius and the lateral head gastrocnemius. These are more commonly called the gastrocs, and they resemble a heart with two long lobes. Then you have the soleus sneaking its way underneath the bellies of the gastrocs. These muscles together are responsible for pointing the toes. The soleus muscle is more hidden and harder to access, and it's more of a stabilizer, as physically it keeps the body from falling forward. Both heads of the gastroc as well as the soleus join onto the Achilles tendon. So too it is a stabilizer on an emotional level. It is the backboard of support and love to the more emotional gastroc muscles.

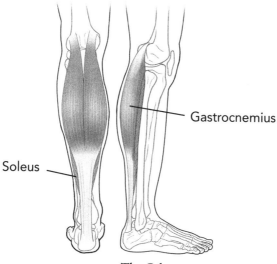

Gastrocnemius

Soleus

The Calves

The gastroc muscles are not just about moving forward in your life. They're more about the heart you put into your actions. When it comes to the calves, they are considered our second heart in our body. It is the calf muscles that contract and pump the blood back up toward our hearts. If your heart's not in it, your calves might give you up. Sometimes calf muscles become sore and stiff simply because you need more salt or more potassium. But other times, your calves get sore and stiff because you are feeling stuck or your heart is simply not in something. It is entirely up to you to ask and determine which it is for you and go from there.

✹ THE CALVES SELF-RELEASE EXERCISE

It is so important to stretch each muscle with intention. Talk to your muscles as you help them remember their true range of motion. These exercises are simple offerings to help you expand your connection to your body. To stretch the calves, simply step back into a deep lunge. Roll the heel down to the ground so that the heel is flat and the calves are stretching. To intensify this stretch and add in the soleus, bend the back knee and bring it down toward the ground, still trying to stretch that heel as close to the floor as you are able. Play with the lunge positions and see which way the calf muscles are able to stretch the most.

The Calf Stretch—Part 1

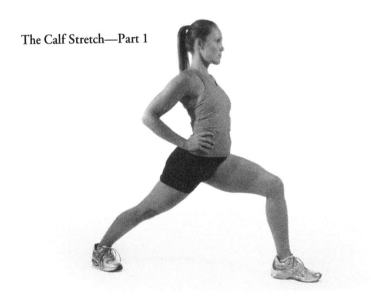

The Calf Stretch—Part 2

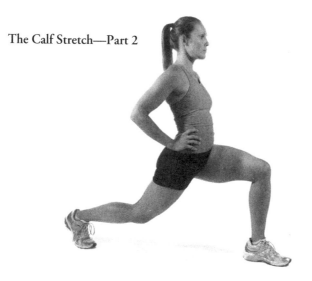

In any stretch that you do for your calves, whether it is simply hanging one foot off a stair and leaning back to stretch the calf or doing downward facing dog or lunges, be sure that you are not only stretching this muscle but talking to this muscle. Working with your calves can help get to the heart of the matter. Thank your calves for the tremendous work that they do. In any massage practice, no matter the size of any person, the calves are always very tender, very sensitive, and quite vulnerable. Give your calves some much needed love with stretch and with intention.

Front of Calves at the Shin Bone: Tibialis Anterior

At the opposite side of the calves on the front side of the body is a muscle that sits right next to the shin bone. That is a kicker of a muscle... literally. This muscle hurts when you do various things, such as kicking. You can really feel an increase in soreness in this muscle if you lift your toes up toward the head (since the action of this muscle both dorsi flexes and inverts the foot). If it hurts when you run on flat pavement, it relieves somewhat with an incline. That muscle is the tibialis anterior, and it is a doozy of a muscle. Tibialis anterior lifts the foot up toward the head, moves it to the side toward the middle of the body, and works with extensor hallucis longus to lift the big toe.

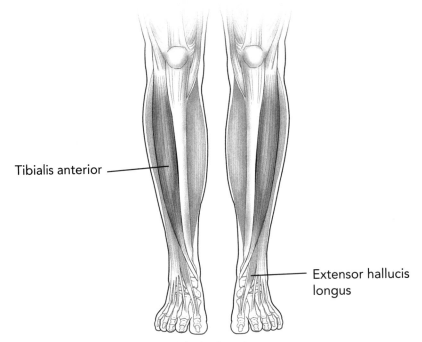

Tibialis anterior

Extensor hallucis longus

Tibialis Anterior

When we get shin splints, this muscle needs to be manually pulled back off the shin bone. It is often extremely painful and holds very intense reactions to being treated. This is a muscle of intensity both physically and emotionally. It is all about things in front of you and movements to get there. Expect some discomfort when working within this area. This is the muscle coming from the lower part of the leg that assists you when you make your decision to move. The hips point, the quads propel, and the tibialis anterior pushes off that big toe and completes the follow through. I have yet to treat an athlete who doesn't carry issues in this muscle. It is not only an emotional muscle but also a highly physical muscle.

❀ THE TIBIALIS ANTERIOR SELF-RELEASE EXERCISE

This is the same stretch that you'll use to release tension in the feet. Sit on your knees with your big toes touching and your ankles as close to each other as you are able to get them. Walk your hands behind your feet and gently lift your knees. Keep your toes tucked under so that your toes are flat on the ground and your heels are facing upward. Use your hands to help you lift the knees.

I knew a yoga teacher once who could rest her bottom in the arches of her feet while doing this stretch. Her knees came fully up into her chest. I will not ask this of you, but keep that image in your head as the feet arch and your bottom is close to that arch as the knees lift up. Feel the stretch throughout the entire front of the lower legs and tops of the feet as well.

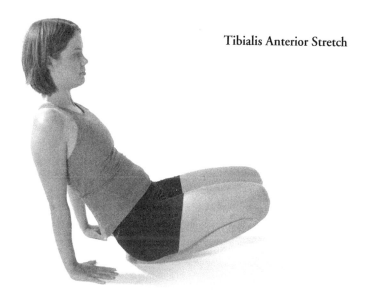

Tibialis Anterior Stretch

This is an easy stretch to bail out of—but don't! It is intense and can border on excruciating, but it works. Talk yourself through it. Be attentive. Hold no less than three deep breaths. Come down slowly and tap the tops of the feet on the ground to relax them after this stretch. This is a tough one! After the stretch, take a moment to connect with your feelings. What lies ahead for you in your immediate future and what movements will you take to get there?

Another physical release you can do yourself to this muscle is to take oil or lotion and rub this part of your leg. Your shin bone runs up and down. It is important to rub side to side to wake this muscle up and give it some much needed attention. Use your thumb or knuckles and do a side to side motion while rubbing before rubbing up and down. Notice the feelings that come up.

Inner/Outer Thighs

The adductor muscles of the inner thighs make the legs close (*adduction* means "to pull into the body"). The abductors of the outer thighs bring the muscles outward, away from the middle of the body. We'll examine both more closely now.

Adductors

The adductor muscles guard your private areas, and they hold a lot of strength and vulnerability. Have you ever pulled your groin? It is a horrible pain. It is intense, it is vulnerable, and it requires true strategy to help treat those muscles involved. The muscles of the inner and outer thighs are gatekeeper muscles. They're very protective over the emotions they hold, so it's important to always be kind when addressing them. This is a supercharged area of the body.

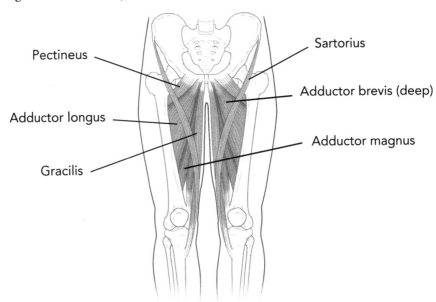

Pectineus

Sartorius

Adductor brevis (deep)

Adductor longus

Adductor magnus

Gracilis

The Adductors—Inner Thighs

The muscles that make up the adductors are: adductor brevis, adductor longus, adductor magnus, gracilis, pectineus, and obturator externus. The adductor muscles of the inner thighs are highly emotional and sensitive, as you can imagine. This allows the legs to stay together or closed. There is so much power in this movement physically and especially emotionally. These muscles have a V shape right at the top of the inner thigh that is one of the endangerment sites in body work. This means it is a site that we mindfully treat physically in massage.

It is, however, one of the areas that we especially treat with lymphatic work. The reason being that in that area is a collection of nerves, veins, arteries, and lymphatics. Going in deep in this area can be damaging and painful. As a muscle area, it needs to be protected and kept safe. This also is the muscle group that guards and keeps safe your private areas. They are the gatekeepers. If you or a client suffered abuse at the hands of another person, they directly overpowered these muscles. These muscles are very sensitive and can easily be hurt in every way imaginable. On the contrary, they also are capable of keeping out unwanted energies or attempts. The emotion to focus on in this space is protection. They are the muscles of protection.

⌘ The Adductor Muscles Self-Release Exercise

This is called the butterfly stretch, and it is used for the adductors. Sitting on the floor, place the bottoms of your feet together, bending your knees and bringing your feet as close in to your body as is comfortable. Before diving down into this stretch, take a deep breath and open your chest and spine. Lift the crown of the head as high up in the air as you are able. Then slightly scoot the bottom back, giving your hips greater access to a forward bend. Bring your nose into the toes and grip the feet with your full hands. Stay in this position no less than ten deep breaths. Allow the hips to open; allow the inner thigh muscles to let go. Bring your knees lower to the ground with each deep breath. You can put your elbows inside the knees to help push the knees down as well. What do you feel when you stretch this area? Are there any feelings of vulnerability that are coming to mind? Explore your emotions and allow any unwanted tension to drift away.

The Butterfly Stretch

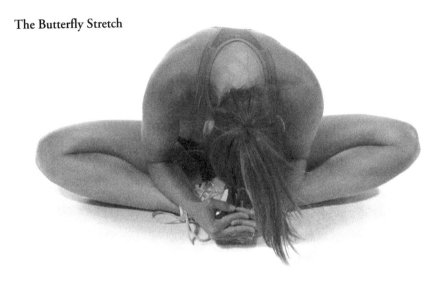

Abductors

The opposite to the adductors are the abductors. These muscles are responsible for moving the legs away from the center line. The muscles that make up the abductors are: piriformis, tensor fasciae latae, sartorius, gluteus medius, and also the gluteus minimus. Also located along the outside of the thighs from the tensor fasciae latae (located high on the pelvic girdle) as well as from gluteus maximus down to below the knee on the lateral condyle of the tibia is a tendon known as the iliotibial band (IT band).

The IT band can wreak havoc if it is tight or injured. Most athletes have really tight IT bands and require great attention to this area. Endurance athletes, runners, and bikers are very prone to IT band syndrome. This is an injury that causes pain along the hip down the side of the leg to just below the knee.

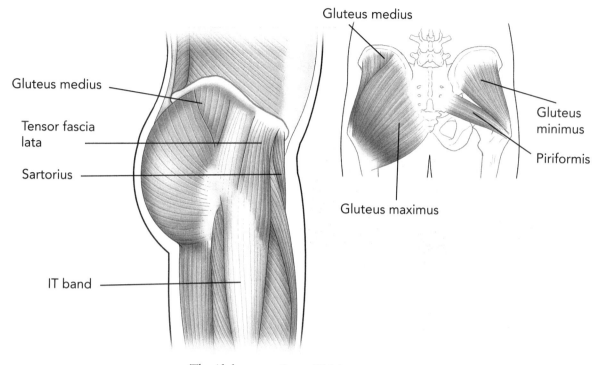

Gluteus medius

Gluteus medius

Tensor fascia lata

Sartorius

IT band

Gluteus minimus

Piriformis

Gluteus maximus

The Abductors—Outer Thighs

It is such a strong band of muscles, tendons, and emotions. When you are in fluid, forward motion energetically, you may be right in line with your IT band. When you feel awkward, running side to side, or overusing not just your body but your mind, this band may cause you to stop and take a second look at your actions and thoughts. You need to be very clear when you set a goal to go for it all the way and trust that you are able to reach it. This is a confidence area. Trust yourself and trust in your ability. Don't second-guess everything, don't let yourself feel lost, and question each decision you are making. If you are in that space, it's time to stop and take a good hard listen within to what you are doing versus what you *want* to be doing. You also need to set the endgame of what you want the goal to look like.

This area of the body does not offer a lot of flexibility physically or emotionally. You need to get very clear on who you are, what you want, and what you are willing to do to get it. Once you set your sights on the goals, never give up on it.

⌘ The Abductor Muscles Self-Release Exercise (Including the IT Band)

The figure four stretch is always a winner for the abductor muscles. It is for when you need to address the abductors, IT bands, and the adductors and have them work in unison. Lying on your back with your knees bent and feet flat on the ground, cross one leg over the other. Now reach your arms around, grabbing with both arms (one from inside the leg and one from outside the bent knee that is on the ground). Pull the leg that is currently on the ground that the other leg is resting on into your chest. Hold this stretch no less than five deep breaths.

Connect with these muscles as you perform the stretch and breathe through each emotion that might arise. This is a time to tap into the energy of these muscles. Talk to them. Do you have a goal in your mind? Are the muscles on board with your goals? Is there exceptional tightness as you stretch and does it loosen up with your deep breaths and communication with it? You must get your body and your mind in line with each other. Be open with your communication in this stretch. This is the time to listen to what your muscles are telling you and let them lead the dialogue.

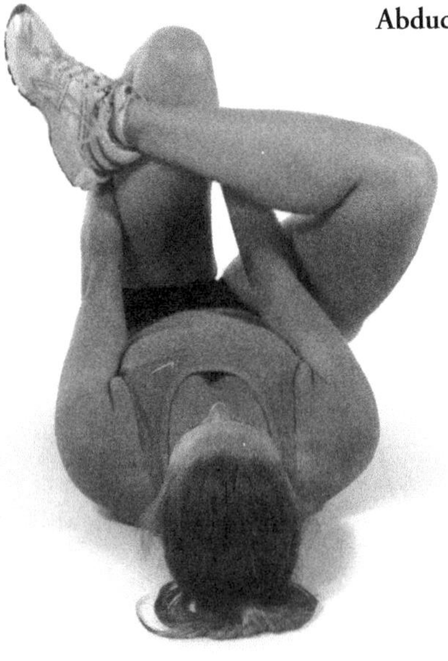

Abductor Stretch—Part 1

Abductor Stretch—Part 2

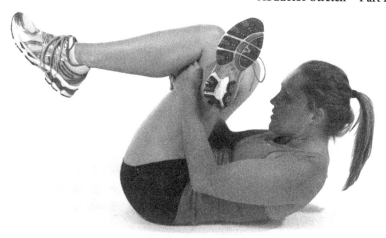

IT Band on Abductor Side

To release tension in the abductors/IT band, the pigeon is an ideal stretch to target these areas, and, as a bonus, it is a huge stretch for the piriformis that we discussed in the glutes chapter. I prefer to begin this stretch from downward facing dog. Bring one leg up toward your hands in a bent position. Walk your hands next to your hips in order to sit upright and then walk your hands out in front of you until they are straight. This will bring relief to the IT band, the abductors, and the piriformis in the most beautiful way.

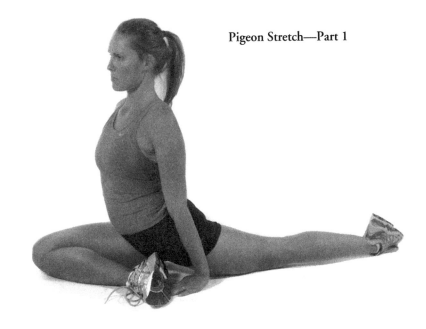

Pigeon Stretch—Part 1

Pigeon Stretch—Part 2

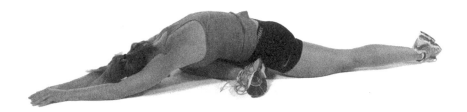

It is not an easy stretch, and likely you will feel resistance in your muscles. They are not quick to relax into this stretch. You must work with yourself and figure out again is this physical, is this emotional, or is this both? Go deep into your body and get to know it on a new level. You deserve to feel freedom from your muscles and your mind.

The Feet and Ankles

The feet as well as the palms of the hands are different from an emotional storehouse. They are instead the maps. They are what takes in the energy from any outside source as well as illustrates their own map from your inside source. They are the keepers of the knowledge and the finders of knowledge.

The muscles of the feet are like the muscles of the hand. On the plantar surface or bottom of the foot the muscles are: the plantar aponeurosis, abductor hallucis, abductor digiti minimi, and the flexor digitorum brevis. The muscles that run deep beneath that layer of superficial muscles are: flexor digiti minimi brevis, adductor hallucis longus, and flexor hallucis brevis. There are abductors and adductors for the big toes and little toes to move them in and out. And the tendons flex and extend the toes. The belly of these muscles that create the movement is also not in the toes (there are no muscles in the toes or ankles) but in the belly of the muscles up in the legs. Tibialis anterior extends the toes up toward the face. The gastrocnemius point the toes and the ankles away from the face toward the ground. There are little muscles within the feet that only attach to the first digit (this is for both in the hands as well and the feet).

The feet are about the path—everything that we have ever experienced shows up on the palms of our hands and on the soles of our feet. In fact, these lines change based on the events in our lives. While standard reflexology of both the feet and the hands are everywhere on the Internet, toe reading is something that only a sacred few do.

Superficial   **Deep Plantar**

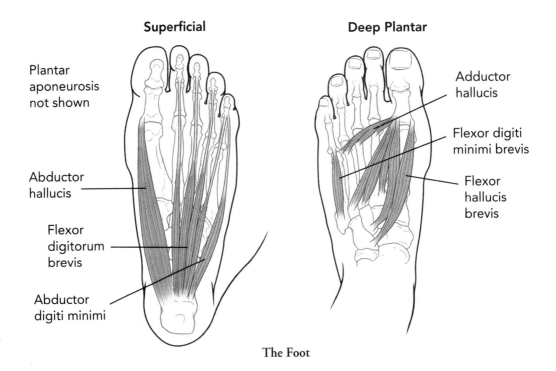

Plantar
aponeurosis
not shown

Adductor
hallucis

Flexor digiti
minimi brevis

Flexor
hallucis
brevis

Abductor
hallucis

Flexor
digitorum
brevis

Abductor
digiti minimi

The Foot

I heard about Cheryl Speen and her toe reading class when I was speaking to the Southwest School of Healing Arts. When I called her, I noticed that my first toe was slightly swollen. I called and left her a message that I was in a writer's block space and was absolutely stuck and that I wanted to interview her for this book to help me open up deeper avenues of understanding. When I talked with her, I told her about my toe. She said, "That makes sense. It's the toe of communication. If you are feeling stuck, it would only make sense to show that to you physically with a little swelling." I had to know more. Please see appendix B for more information from Cheryl on toe reading as well as ankles and feet. As a side note, after I spoke with her I was totally jazzed and my writer's block lifted. The following morning, I noticed that my first toe had also returned to its regular size and shape. Coincidence? I think not.

❀ THE FEET AND ANKLES SELF-RELEASE EXERCISE

This stretch is best done following the stretch for the anterior tibialis. Once you have done the first stretch, stay in the kneeling position. Sitting on your heels, come forward onto your hands to get your feet in the correct position. Tuck the toes flat on the floor and the pads of your feet flat to the floor. Now try to sit up on your heels. This stretch is serious. It stretches the myofascial tendon running down the arch of the foot as well as all of the muscles in the feet. Do not bail out of this stretch. It is hard, but you can do it! Breathe at least three deep breaths into this stretch. It is easy to let your mind race and wonder in trying to do this difficult stretch, but the purpose is to link your mind to your feet and get clear and powerful with your intentions.

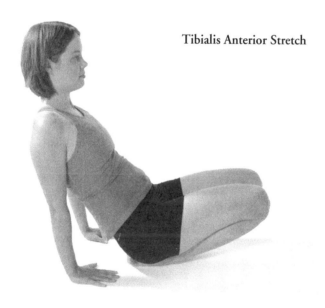

Tibialis Anterior Stretch

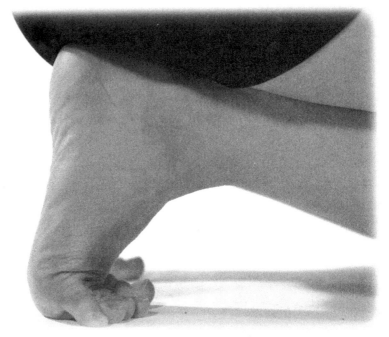

The Tibialis Anterior Stretch and Foot Stretch—Part 1

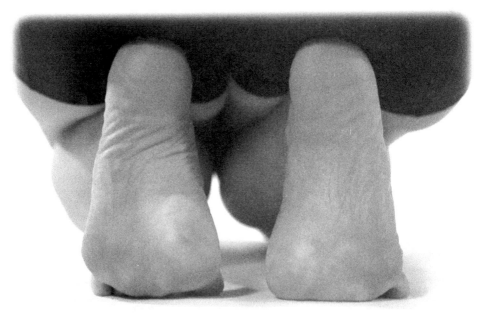

The Tibialis Anterior Stretch and Foot Stretch—Part 2

Affirmations

When you engage in the self-release exercise, you are targeting the specific muscle group. Adding in the affirmation at the same time connects the body with the mind and strengthens your intentions for the highest outcome. For every affirmation, choose one or more statement that best fits where you are currently or create your own. Repeat the statement throughout the day.

Focus your thoughts on your feet, your legs, and the information that is coming from them. As you do so, you might think of this affirmation and see how the energy in your feet and legs respond.

- I am *able.*
- I am moving in the direction of my goals.
- I am able to run free and move my body in alignment with my heart and mind.
- I am an open conduit for love and forward motion in my life.
- I am strong, and I am powerful.
- I trust my path.

⌘ Spoon Technique for Stimulating the Feet

I chose this particular self-exercise tool to stimulate the energy centers of the feet. You can do this in the morning or at night, and I encourage you to do this to your children and friends as well. There was a man who tested this particular practice on his children. He bought several metal spoons, created a foot mat with them, and put it inside the door for the children to step on as they entered the house (after they removed their shoes). The day the children stepped onto the mat, they came inside, sat right at the table, and proceeded to do their homework without issue. He thought *This can't be true!* He decided to have the children enter the home through the back door the next day and not use the mat. When prompted to sit at the table, the children both put up a stink about sitting down to do homework. He began to share this spoon technique to help others stimulate the feet because so many meridians begin and end in the feet. Here is the exercise with the metal spoon:

Use the back of a metal spoon to make small circles and figure eights all along your entire foot. Start around the back of the heel, making small circles or small figure eights. Work across the heels, over and around them, moving your way side to side upward to the arch and so on until you circle over the tops of each toe. Notice the energy in the foot that you have just done this exercise to. Notice the energy emanating from the sole of that foot. Notice the difference between that foot and the one that you have not yet treated. Then treat the other foot to match the energy. Close your eyes afterward and feel the energy in your feet. Notice whatever sensations come into your mind and into your thoughts. Feel the open energy through the feet in this moment. Using the metal spoon stimulates these energy centers and grounds your body at the same time.

Suggested Stones for the Legs, Feet, and Ankles

Amazonite: A wonderful stone to use to help move forward and embrace new adventures.

Hematite: The ultimate grounding stone. This stone is wonderful to wear around the ankles to keep you grounded and rooted deeply.

Watermelon tourmaline: A stone for relieving stresses as you move into new phases of life and providing security and clarity in your decisions to move.

Suggested Essential Oils for the Legs, Feet, and Ankles

Black pepper oil: Is great for the ankles.

Frankincense: Is the ideal oil for grounding and earth energy.

Peppermint, eucalyptus, rosemary, spearmint: Are all great oils to mix and match for the leg muscles. These help ease muscle soreness. Do not use these directly on the skin; they must be diluted with a carrier oil.

❀ Moving Meditation Practice

Go outside and take your shoes and socks off. Stand with your legs hip width apart and dig your bare feet deeply into the earth. Spread your toes and feel the ground beneath you. Connect yourself into earth energy. Open your foot receptors and connect the earth energy and your body energy through every pore of your feet. As you stand strong, balanced, and steady, give thought to where you are in this exact moment of your life. Give thought to the things that may be holding you back from going after your dreams. If it's all the mind chatter of the responsibilities you are faced with, please just for this moment, move those thoughts out of your mind. Put them safely in a box, close the top, and move it out of the living area of your mind for now. Think more of the life you choose. Who are you? What do you love? Are you pursuing in any part your passions? Feel not just your feet but your ankles. Ask yourself "Am I enjoying life?" Feel your calves and ask yourself "Is my heart in it?" (Whatever *it* is to you). Feel your knees and ask yourself "Am I feeling stuck? Am I able to move into the next phase of what I want for my life?" Feel your quads and your hamstrings and ask yourself "What direction is the next step for me?" Then, ever so mindfully, begin to walk softly among the grass or dirt or rocks that are in your area. Feel the elements beneath your toes and heels. Walk with purpose and intention. Do not step on flowers, do not harm anything beneath you. Notice, if you are in grass, how heavy your footprint is into the grass. Can you lighten up your steps? Can you lighten your load in this walk? Can you lighten your load in your mind? Can you lighten your load in your life?

Chapter 7

The Abdominal Muscles, Diaphragm, and the Psoas
Your Storehouse for Where the Real Vulnerability Lives

The abdominal muscles play the role of support, both physically and emotionally. Not only do they allow you to stand upright, working in conjunction with the back muscles to help keep you strong and stable but it also protects the colon, intestines, and many other vital organs. They also play a huge role in assisting with emotional processing and releasing. The rectus abdominis, internal/external obliques, and the transversus abdominis are mighty muscles that cover the entirety of the abdominal area. Notice if you have a really good, deep belly laugh that you will feel sore in the whole stomach. This is because these muscles are connected to your emotion. If you've ever had that bend over, cry your eyes out, and can't even function kind of cry, you may have noticed that these muscles will be sore for days on end.

The abdominal muscles do not hold on to emotional trauma in the same way that the psoas does. The psoas runs through your abdominal region, and it is arguably the second most emotional muscle in the body after the longus colli. We'll talk about the psoas later on in this chapter, as it's very different from the other muscles in this area. As emotions are processed through the organs, the psoas, and the very sacred vulnerable reproductive areas, the abdominal muscles provide additional strength, power, and protection—they help with release, they support, they assist, but they do not hold on to and store the emotional energy in the way that other muscles do. The abdominal muscles are the protectors. It's what lies underneath that really bears the brunt of emotional stress.

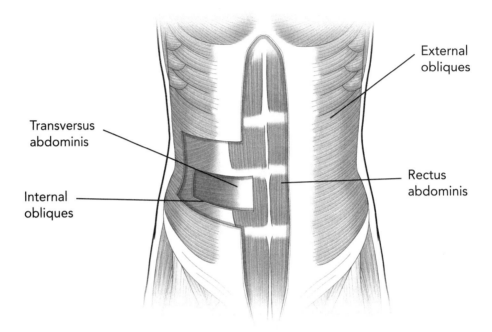

Transversus abdominis

Internal obliques

External obliques

Rectus abdominis

The Abdominal Muscles

Most mammals walk with their abdominal sections facing downward toward the ground, as they walk on all fours. We as humans have this part of ourselves fully exposed out into the world. Before even getting into the energetics and emotions of these areas, the physical vulnerability of the abdomen is easy to realize. A hit to the stomach affects the stomach, the colon, the large and small intestines, the spleen, the liver, and the gallbladder! All of those things are tucked away into the soft part of the abdominal region. Plus the pancreas that hides just behind the stomach. Then you have your lungs and heart protected by your ribs, but those also can easily be hurt physically by any amount of force to these areas. Almost all of your vital organs are housed right there in the softest, most vulnerable area of your body. That is a lot to carry around exposed to the world.

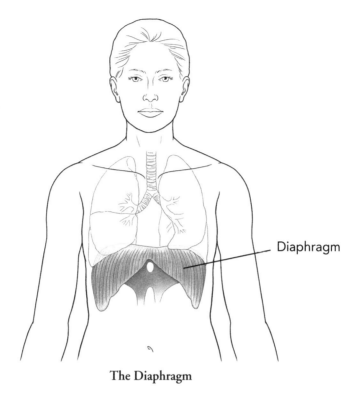

Diaphragm

The Diaphragm

The diaphragm muscle is also an important piece of this puzzle. This muscle is not an abdominal muscle, and it does not carry the same emotional energy that the abdominals do. It is not a deep hip flexor the way the psoas is. It is its own unique muscle with its own energy. I once worked on someone who had a collapsed diaphragm. It was utterly painful to work on someone who could barely catch a breath. The muscle was hardened and atrophied. Both the hypochondriac and empath parts of me didn't know what to do with myself when my hands touched that area! It hurt me to feel such a breakdown of such a mighty muscle. The diaphragm is responsible in the largest part for our breath. The diaphragm is responsible for 80 percent of our entire lung capacity.

The diaphragm is the place where your intuition is stored. It is a place where deep strength and trust emanate out into the entire being. We are often reminded to breathe deeply from our diaphragm. We are reminded to stand up straight and pull from our diaphragm for strength, posture, poise, and confidence. It is the place deep within where we find our true voice. The diaphragm holds a very magical key to our self-worth and our trust in our own judgment. This muscle is profound and stoic in its emotional nature. If you want to capture and cultivate the essence of who you really are, what you stand for, how you value your own worth, and how you use your voice to echo all of this—the diaphragm is where you will find it.

An activity to help you become united with your diaphragm is *pranayama*—the breath of life. We discuss *pranayama* later in this book. (See appendix A for a full description and a variety of breathing techniques.)

An easy exercise to connect to the diaphragm is to place one hand just above the navel (below the ribs) and the other hand on the center of your chest. Exhale fully and with intention. Inhale and lift the navel away from the spine. Exhale and bring the navel toward the spine. Do not move the chest—notice your hand on your belly rises and falls with your breath. The hand on your chest should not move. This isolates the diaphragm muscle. Repeat this practice.

That's a lot of emotional possibilities, and we haven't even gone into the deeper muscles and what they carry! Plus, you also have the reproductive organs that lie in the second chakra and the gut emotions that lie in the third chakra. The reproductive organs can store the emotional memories of a lifetime of celebrations and disappointments and worse...any trauma that was at the hands of someone else that you experienced can potentially be stored in this area. Many cancers are associated with these body parts. The muscle that lies directly in this path is the psoas. The energy sits in the chakras, the emotions pair with the meridians, and the pains and traumas sit in the belly of the psoas. All aspects must be addressed and treated for a release that can change the path.

⌘ The Abdominals Self-Release Exercise

Rub the belly to cover all of the organs. Rub your belly in the direction of the colon so that you help the flow of the energy release and do not constipate your body. Place your right hand on the stomach and rest the left hand on top of the right hand. Bring your hands up to the top right of your stomach, just below the ribs. Begin from the top right, circling over to the left side, down the left side, and back up to the right side. Circle left to right clockwise. Imagine your body as a clock, where your head is 12, your left side is 3, your pubic bone is 6, and your right side is 9. Rub in this direction with intention and love in your hands. Try to make the circle at least three times.

Think about your internal organs and connect with this area as you do this exercise. Talk to your body and listen as it responds. In the concept of meridians, the organs are paired with an emotion. The emotions that are associated with the organs in this area are:

Organ	Out of Balance	Balanced
Bladder	Anxiety/futility	Hope
Gallbladder	Anger/rage/judgment	Tolerant/kind
Heart	Heartache	Love
Kidney	Fear/shame	Gentleness
Large intestine	Controlling	Release/trust
Liver	Anger/rage	Acceptance
Lungs	Sadness	Inspiration
Pericardium	Overwhelm	Balance
Small intestine	Scattered/divided	Unity/balance
Spleen/pancreas	Excessive thinking/worry	Congruency/impartiality
Triple warmer	Fight, flight, or freeze	Secure

The Psoas

The iliopsoas, more commonly known as the psoas, has been referred to as the seat of the soul or the muscle of the soul. It's one of the most important core-stabilizing muscles. The psoas is a deep hip flexor muscle that originates from the lumbar spine and joins with iliacus and inserts way high up on the lesser trochanter—the tiny notch on the upper inner part of the femur bone in the leg. The belly of the psoas runs between the hip bone and the pubic bone. It also connects to the diaphragm and is associated with breathing functions.

When it comes to the psoas muscle there is so much information out there on every level physically, clinically, emotionally, and spiritually. Physically the muscle is the only one in the body that crosses from the back of the body to the front of the body. This muscle also has an integration with the lumbar plexus, which is its link to the central nervous system and deep emotion. Liz Koch, author of *The Psoas Book* and also *Core Awareness* among other books and articles regarding the psoas, is considered a psoas guru in many circles. She says:

> Although the psoas has been thought to serve the spine as a guide wire creating stabilization, its main job is to message subtle changes in weight, location, and safety. The psoas bridges the belly enteric brain, central, nervous system, and autonomic nervous systems. The large nerve ganglion located within the belly core going to the digestive and reproductive organs passes over, embeds into, and through the psoas. Serving as messenger of the core, our psoas translates and transmits all expressions of safety, harmony, and integrity; signaling whether or not we are centered and congruent or encumbered and vulnerable.

The psoas is a sacred muscle that holds a lot of emotion. Fear, stress, anxiety, emotional trauma, physical trauma—all this energy can present itself in the psoas.

The psoas muscle is linked to the autonomic nervous system (sympathetic and parasympathetic, aka the fight, flight, or freeze response). The fight, flight, or freeze reflexes of the body are all propelled through the psoas. If you fight, you have to get up, power off, and go into the fight. That begins in the core of the body, specifically the psoas muscle. The flight aspect, having to get up and make a run for it, also comes from that same place. The freeze reflex usually ends with a person lying down in a fetal position, scared to death, and can do nothing but drop. If you curl up in a ball, you are bringing the knees toward the chest. The psoas is the muscle that brings that movement to life. This muscle is strong, powerful, forceful, and fully able to move you in any direction in your life. Not only is it strong and full of power but emotionally it holds for you the deepest experiences of your life.

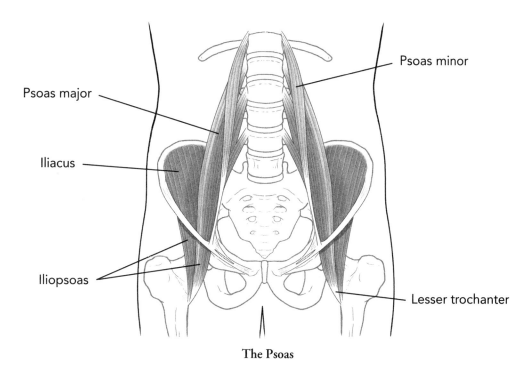

The Psoas

Think about this: Your ears are the gatherers of information, your eyes are the hunter, and your hips are the movers. Your hips propel the direction of your next move, and the muscle that enables that move is the psoas. When making any decision in life, you gather your information (listen for cues and collect your thoughts), you set the target and create your goal (set your sights on the next goal to reach), and you activate the psoas and move your hips and then activate the legs and feet toward that goal. The psoas muscle is deep in the body, and it holds many secrets about you. It is a record keeper.

Physically this is a muscle that can hold every tension. It also tightens up if your legs have been overly bent and locked up for too long. Sitting in a chair, whether in an office or in a car, for long periods of time, directly affects this muscle. This is the muscle that locks up as you stand up and it feels like your back is about to go out—it's the psoas! It is my opinion that any emotional components that might be surrounding the reproductive organs also sit in the belly of the psoas muscle.

Releasing physical and emotional tension in this muscle can be extremely painful, but the psoas is a major player for the entire body and taking care of it is essential. The psoas is the gateway into good back health, strong hip health, and a bridge to the emotional health. Having this muscle treated and released properly provides enormous benefits to any athlete who overworks this area, to any person carrying around the energy of unresolved or unhealed trauma, and to anyone who suffers from a low back injury. When the psoas is healthy, we are more stable emotionally as well as physically, and the energy within our bodies can flow more freely.

Treating the psoas through physical techniques such as massage requires professional training. Unless you have professional training and you know what you're doing, do not attempt to treat this area whatsoever. Go to a licensed physical therapist or a massage therapist and make sure they have the right certifications and training to treat the psoas. Caution is needed because treating the psoas requires attentiveness, skill, and precision. If the person giving the massage does not pay close enough attention to the placement of their hands in finding the psoas, it could have negative consequences elsewhere, such as perforation of the colon. In fact, some massage schools are completely opting out of teaching this complex and delicate work due to the difficulty and the risks involved. In my opinion, this is a shame. For massage schools to devalue the emphasis that this muscle has on the back and lower body, the emotional body, and the vulnerable body itself… this should be taught to every single person who does body work in any school. Period. The psoas is more often than not the key to releasing discomfort in the low back, and yet it is frequently overlooked. On the other side of the equation, there are full books written on the psoas muscle alone. I can only hope that the depth to which I am expressing my own heartfelt appreciation and awe of this muscle comes through appropriately in this relatively short overview. Get to know your psoas.

There are stretches and other techniques that anyone can do for the psoas to help release the tension it holds and to support the muscle's overall health and function.

❀ The Psoas Self-Release Exercise

To stretch the psoas on your own, start by lying on the edge of your bed. Have the edge of your bottom at the very edge of the bed. Then lay back. Put one foot down on the ground and hug the other bent knee/leg into your chest. The leg that is hanging down toward the ground should be bent. If the knee of the long leg can go lower than the plane of your hip bones, your psoas muscle is not too tight. If you are unable to drop the long knee down lower than your hip level, you have an issue. This is a great stretch for the muscle as well. (The first photo is the starting point and second photo is the stretch.)

The Psoas Stretch—Part 1

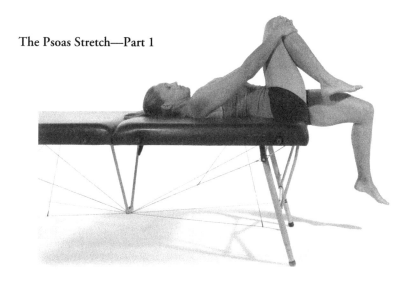

The Psoas Stretch—Part 2

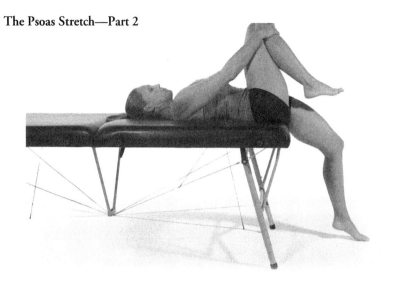

The other way to stretch is to lie on your stomach and pull the heels up to the buttocks. If you can, put a small pillow or rolled towel underneath your bent knee to get a little more out of the stretch.

Affirmations

When you engage in the self-release exercise, you are targeting the specific muscle group. Adding in the affirmation at the same time connects the body with the mind and strengthens your intentions for the highest outcome. For every affirmation, choose one or more statement that best fits where you are currently or create your own. Repeat the statement throughout the day.

- I am *safe now*.
- I am secure.
- I affirm that my body is healthy, and I am in rhythm with my body.
- I go with the flow and not against it.
- I trust my gut to lead me to the highest outcome possible.

- I am strong in my body and in my thoughts.
- I trust. I am in the flow. I believe in *me*.

❀ AN INVITATION TO COMMUNICATE WITH YOUR RECORD KEEPER

Lie down with your knees bent and your feet on the ground. Place your hands on your lower stomach between the hip bones and the pubic bones. There lies your psoas muscle. As you breathe into this space, feel the energy beneath your hands. Don't go digging trying to find this muscle because I don't want you to do any damage. Although if you are the kind of person who doesn't listen to this advice and goes digging, at least know that as you lift your leg, the psoas will present itself to you if you are of a leaner stature. It's not about the actual muscle location here though, it's about the energy that you might find beneath your hand knowing it is somewhere above the muscle. Use both hands, one on each side over the area for best results.

Close your eyes and breathe with intention into this space. Talk to this muscle. Introduce yourself to it if you haven't ever before. Let this area of yourself know that you are now going to make an effort to be in alignment with it and not against it if you might have been in the past. As you keep your eyes closed and your hands over the area, ask this area to reveal itself to you. Ask for this muscle to introduce itself to you as well. Notice if any strange images come into your mind. Do you see any old memories? Do strange people that you don't think about come up for you? Do colors come into play for you here? Only you know the language of your body so only you will know what the messages are that might be coming through to you. Linking into the psoas is akin to dream interpretation. Only you can truly tap into what your dreams might be telling you, so is the same with this muscle. You may want to tell it that you are sorry for not listening to it before now. You may want to let it know that if there are emotions being kept there, that you are now strong enough to handle them and they can give them back to you to take care of and release.

Breathe deeply and intentionally with each breath as you hold your hands over this space and tune your mind into this area. Ask that this muscle release to you its pains, its tension, and its secrets. You are now strong enough to handle it and it doesn't need to hold so many memories anymore in there. Take anything that comes into your mind as a message and work with the potential images, not against anything by second-guessing this process. This is not a guided meditation, it is a guided invitation and the rest is up to you. Please do take the time to go there. You won't regret it.

Suggested Stones for Abdominal Muscles and the Psoas

Girasol opals: These stones help you to get in touch with your inner truth. In working with getting down deep into what really is the issue, these are fantastic stones to have in each hand of the person doing the deeper dive within. This stone has many healing abilities but this is the primary use for these stones for myself and my clients because I have found no other stone that can pull the magic out like a girasol opal can. Consider these the truth-telling stones.

Moonstone: A powerful stone that helps support the reproductive organs, the second chakra, and the psoas muscle.

Rose quartz: Always a smart option because of its intensely loving energy. For this area that is so vulnerable, use the rose quartz as often as you are able.

Turquoise: A deep healer that matches incredibly well in this area. Lay a turquoise right over the muscle as you do the invitation for the gatekeeper meditation work.

Suggested Essential Oils for the Abdominal Muscles and the Psoas

I would go with the deep grounders for this area.

Frankincense: Always a smart grounder, and it also connects you to the higher realms of energy. Use this oil in your meditations for not only grounding but also for the connecting of heaven and earth. Combine with myrrh to add the highest amounts of energy to your meditation experiences.

Patchouli: A top choice for me for grounding and earth energy while you learn this new part of your body. This area is already so high in vibration, you need something to keep you to the earth.

Sandalwood: Also gives you that earthy vibration.

⌘ Connecting to Your Sacred Light Visualization

Deep within you is a small flame of light. Like a candle newly lit, look at the flame inside yourself. See this light as a small flame deep within your lower body from the second chakra and reproductive area. Look into this little flame of light. With each breath, watch as this little flame begins to expand. Ever so slightly with each breath you take, the light within you expands—the light becomes bigger and bigger and bigger and expands within your entire being. Now your entire being is filled with this great white light. Take another deep breath in and out and allow the light to explode from your being, now surrounding you from the outside in a gigantic white flame of light, of heat, of vitality, of renewal, and of radiant health. Continue to breathe deeply into this light, let the light become you. Bask in the loving kindness that is the light from your own being. This is your divine light. This is your birthright. This light has always been yours and can always be yours. Call upon this light any time you need healing and reminding of the greatness that you are.

We ask that in this moment all cells, all molecules, all parts of your body, and your DNA be corrected, recomposed, and restored to perfect harmony. All cells in your body are now healthy, and all cells that were not healthy fall away outside of your light into the earth to be recycled and renewed. I ask that in this space you feel the lightness and perfection of harmonious health and a calm, positive, loving mind.

Be at peace and be of service both to yourself and to others. Understand and accept the sacred unity of *you* in this moment. Share this version of yourself with the world. You don't have to turn your light down just because you finish with this visualization. Stay within your light and be mindful of it as often as you are able.

In this moment, you are able to experience perfect health and harmony.

Chapter 8

The Arms, Shoulders, and Hands

Your Storehouse for Embracing Love and Claiming Vitality

The arms, hands, and shoulders are associated with embracing life, people, and situations. In this chapter, you'll learn about the emotional energies that are stored in these frequently used muscles. Your arms deal with pushing and pulling, accepting and rejecting, and embracing or repelling.

The biceps embrace, bring in, and give more affection, while the triceps push back, stabilize, and protect. The forearms are more associated with the throat and neck. In fact, singers are taught to massage their forearms just before performing so that the vocal chords will be in prime condition, as there are energy lines that connect the forearm muscles directly with the muscles of the throat. The shoulder muscles are where we carry burdens, and you're likely to get tight in this area if you are type A personality or have trouble surrendering control, insisting that you can do whatever it is much better than whoever else. The elbows are associated with our ability or inability to change directions with ease, and the wrists also represent movement and ease. The stress of repetitive movements will also be shown in the wrists as well as the forearms, and these physical causes should never be ignored, even as you explore the emotional aspects.

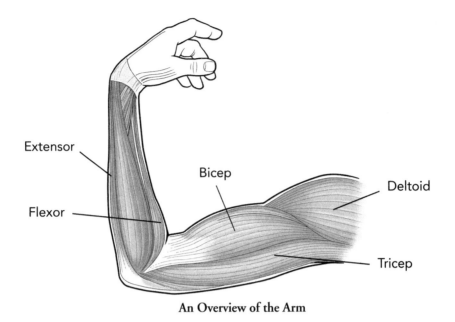

An Overview of the Arm

Embracing life, embracing the new, hugging, holding—these are all in the arms. The opposite is also part of the emotional storehouse within the arms—resisting, pushing away, holding back, and protection.

Deltoid (Shoulders)

The deltoid is one large muscle with three distinct fiber directions (anterior, middle, and posterior) that make up the triangle-shaped musculature at the top of the arm. The movement of the deltoid is: anterior, flexion, and medial rotation; middle, abduction; posterior, lateral rotation, and extension.

Emotionally, the deltoids deal with embracing just the way the arms do, but they also deal heavily with the emotions of carrying extra baggage. Whatever extra baggage you have been carrying around, it must be physically and emotionally picked up and carried. Imagine a heavy bag that you have been keeping with you and each time you are treated poorly, put down, embarrassed, put off, or pushed away, you add another piece to your baggage and continue to pick it up and carry it off with you everywhere you go.

This emotionally heavy load is often physically stored as tension in the muscles of the shoulders. Many people have serious tears or aches in their shoulders that have resulted from overuse or injury, but there can often be an emotional component to the pain felt in these powerful muscles. If you're having trouble with your deltoids, ask yourself if you might be carrying around any extra heavy baggage such as guilt, shame, sadness, or fear.

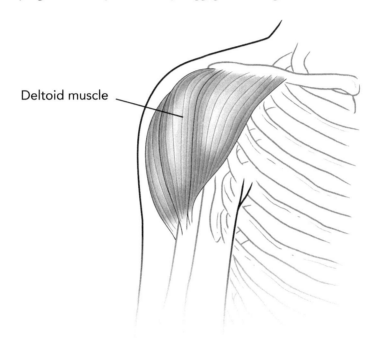

Deltoid muscle

The Deltoid Muscle

On the brighter side, because the deltoids move a ball and socket, like the ball and socket in the femur of the thigh, the arms can move in full circle motions. Therefore, there is not just a pushing up, pushing out, protection, or acceptance for the body in this area. Giving, receiving, protecting, and redirecting all exists within the shoulders. Feeling the weight of the world on the hard days or feeling the weightless love of receiving it and holding on tight are emotions that both exist here.

� THE DELTOIDS SELF-RELEASE EXERCISE

Downward facing dog is the absolute best shoulder stretch there is. Start on your hands and knees, place the palms flat on the floor in front of you. Angle your thumbs to face each other and your middle fingers to face straight ahead. Keep the palms of the hands flat to the floor. Bring your bottom up high, straighten the legs, and walk the feet back until you are in an upside down V position with your bottom being the tip of the V. Arch slightly in your lower back and push your body weight over your heels and not so much in your arms and shoulders. Allow your head to be heavy and match the ears to the shoulders or below. Keep trying to lift your bottom higher and higher and lower your heels flat into the floor. You can have your feet hip-width apart, a few inches apart, or touching. Hold this pose at least ten breaths for great release.

Downward Facing Dog

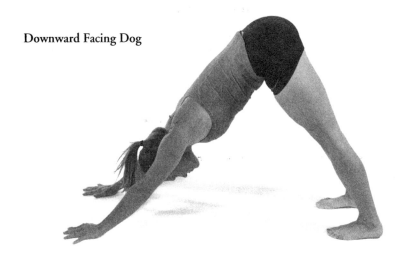

Affirmations

When you engage in the self-release exercise, you are targeting the specific muscle group. Adding in the affirmation at the same time connects the body with the mind and strengthens your intentions for the highest outcome. For every affirmation, choose one or more statement that best fits where you are currently or create your own. Repeat the statement throughout the day.

- I am *strong*.
- I am supple, and I am able to defend my life, my positions, and my beliefs.
- I allow negativity to roll off me.
- I embrace the really great offerings of life.
- I embrace my body, my heart, and my life.

Biceps

When we hug someone, we open our arms out wide to embrace them and pull them in close to our hearts. Grabbing hold of something and bringing it in toward your heart space is the magic of the arms and hands. The optimal energy flow of the biceps muscles is open, loving, and enveloping. When the biceps are having issues, we might want to look and see if there may be an emotional component to the breakdown. Are you wanting to embrace something that is simply not there? Are you open to something in particular but not getting what you want to have? These emotions will reveal themselves in the flexors, both in the forearm and within the biceps.

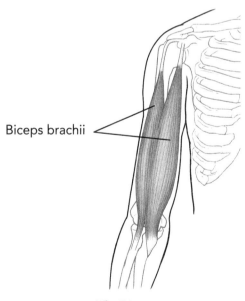

Biceps brachii

The Biceps

The bicep muscles have two lobes to the muscle. Think of it like a long heart shape with the two lobes of the heart toward the elbow side and the connection of the one point of the heart right in the high shoulder area. Like the calves that are also heart shaped, this muscle is the heart of the arms and carries with it that same sort of emotion. Embracing life, loving your life, or, on the other side when people experience things like bicep tears, you might wonder if your heart isn't into something.

⌘ The Biceps Self-Release Exercise

The doorway stretch is done by taking one or both hands inside the doorway and walk forward until your arms are straight and your chest is open and you feel the stretch in the biceps.

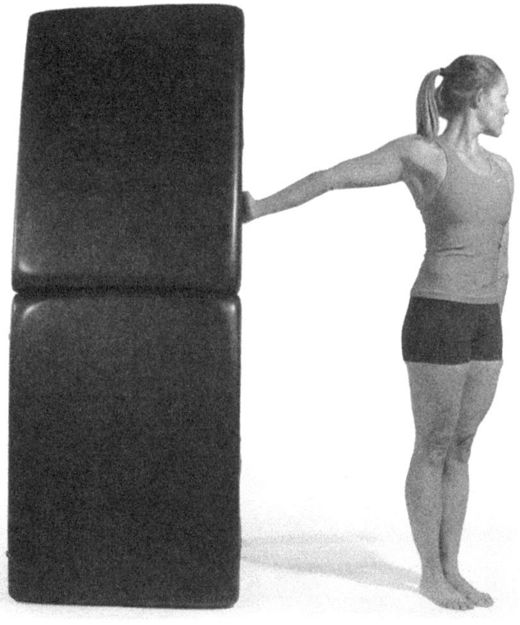

Doorway Stretch

The Triceps

The triceps consist of three muscles and the physical use is to push away from the body. The biceps bend the arms and the triceps straighten them back out. This is a push muscle, both physically as well as emotionally. The triceps help to push out what is not needed. They also repel, protect, and enforce whatever we need them to enforce. They are strong muscles and they protect not just our physical sphere, but our energetic sphere as well. When you're having problems with the triceps, it might be helpful to examine the protective emotions you may be storing in these muscles. Are you feeling especially resistant? Are you fully allowing the happiness and success you wish for to enter your life? Are you feeling out of control or overwhelmed? Examining your feelings can help you get to the root of the problem so that you can release these energies and relax the muscle. Issues in the elbow or shoulder can also manifest as tension in the triceps, so you might want to look into these areas, as well.

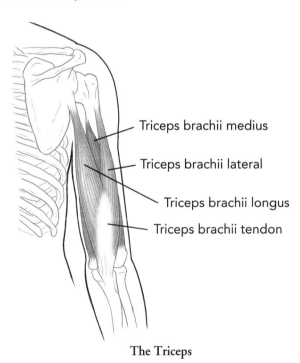

Triceps brachii medius

Triceps brachii lateral

Triceps brachii longus

Triceps brachii tendon

The Triceps

⌘ The Triceps Self-Release Exercise

Simply giving yourself a hug is what can stretch these muscles. It also brings the love inside to your heart space, using both the biceps and the triceps to make this happen. Self-love is so important to healing. This simple self-release stretch can be so special if you close your eyes and let the love in and circle through you.

The Self-Hug Stretch

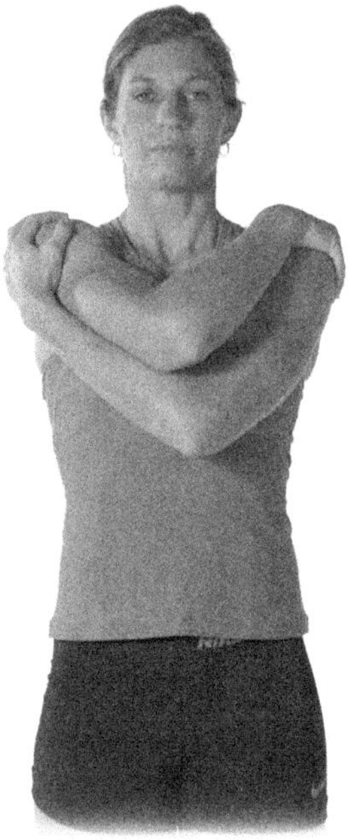

Flexors

The forearm flexors are your grippers. They grab hold of what you want and hang on tight! They also pull the fingers in toward the hand to hold something. They also bend the wrist. Flexors are strong muscles that emotionally help you to hold your ground. Grab ahold of your feelings, your wants, and your needs and trust in your own ability to get them. If you want something bad enough, you will make it happen. If you don't, you make excuses. Make sure these muscles are being worked!

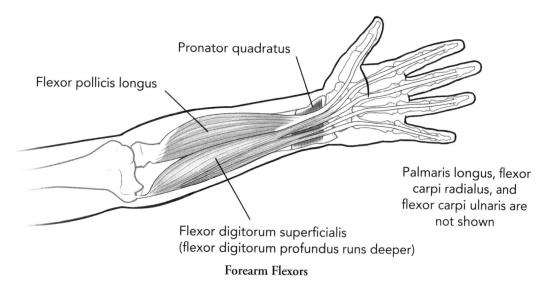

Pronator quadratus

Flexor pollicis longus

Palmaris longus, flexor carpi radialus, and flexor carpi ulnaris are not shown

Flexor digitorum superficialis
(flexor digitorum profundus runs deeper)

Forearm Flexors

⌘ The Flexors Self-Release Exercise

Extend one arm out in front of you with the fingertips facing up. Your knuckles should be facing you and the palm away from the body. Place the other hand over your palm and fingers, covering both areas so you are not just pulling the fingers back. Use the back hand to pull the whole hand and fingers toward your face. This stretches the flexors of the forearms.

Flexors Stretch

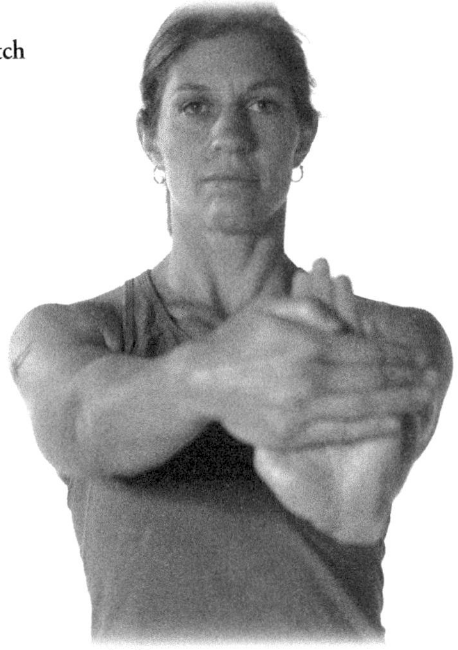

Affirmations

When you engage in the self-release exercise, you are targeting the specific muscle group. Adding in the affirmation at the same time connects the body with the mind and strengthens your intentions for the highest outcome. For every affirmation, choose one or more statement that best fits where you are currently or create your own. Repeat the statement throughout the day.

- I am open to receiving life's many bountiful blessings.
- I am worthy to receive.
- I stand with my arms open, my chest open, and my heart open to receive blessings and goodness. I am free to choose happiness.
- I allow myself to feel good and experience joy.

Extensors

The extensors are the muscles on the knuckle side of the forearms. Extensors extend or straighten. The extensor muscles include the extensor side of the forearms, which is the knuckle side of the hands. While the flexor side is about bringing energies in toward the body, embracing, allowing and opening, gripping and holding on, the extensor side is all about pushing out, resisting, and protecting.

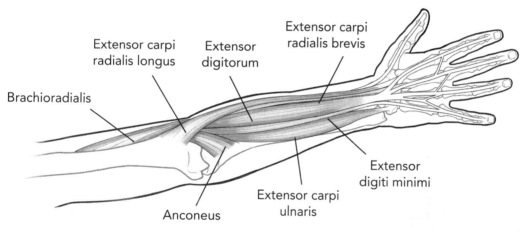

The Extensor Muscles

⌘ The Extensors Self-Release Exercise

Coming from the previous stretch of the forearm flexors. Turn the fingers down toward the ground. Place the other hand on the outside of the knuckles and hand. Pull gently the whole hand and fingers toward your body. This stretches the forearm extensors.

Extensors Stretch

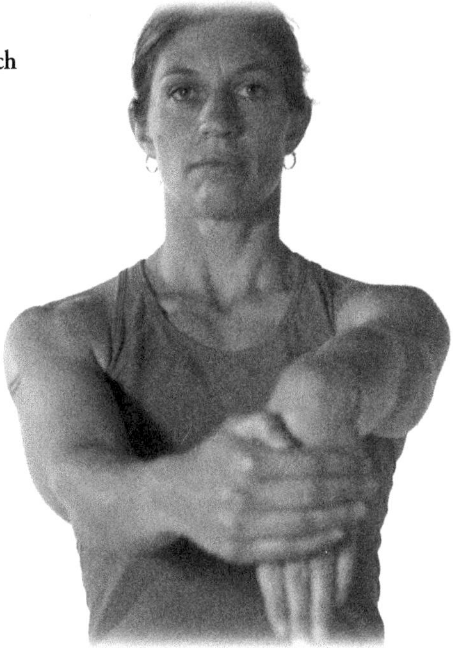

Affirmations

When you engage in the self-release exercise, you are targeting the specific muscle group. Adding in the affirmation at the same time connects the body with the mind and strengthens your intentions for the highest outcome. For every affirmation, choose one or more statement that best fits where you are currently or create your own. Repeat the statement throughout the day.

- I am balanced and stable.
- I am strong, and I only allow things to enter my field that are for my highest good and greatest joy.
- I resist negativity in my field now.
- I grab hold of the good things in my life.

Elbows and Wrists

The elbows and the wrists are both associated with changing directions and with how we allow or resist vulnerability and fluidity within those movements. Flexibility in change is the key to the joints in the arms. If you're having trouble with your elbows or wrists, look at your emotions surrounding flexibility, change, and vulnerability.

Are you resisting something? Is there something that has become too close for comfort? Are you trying to rearrange and struggling to do so? Are you the person responsible for holding down the fort, and is it getting to be a bit much? These are things to look further into to understand issues in the wrists and elbows.

Forearm Flexors and Extensors and Repetitive Motion Issues

When it comes to the forearms, repetitive motion issues are the number one complaint. Carpal tunnel syndrome, tennis elbow, and golfer's elbow are very common. We use our hands, wrists, and forearms all the time, and very rarely do we stop to stretch them, check in on them, and connect them to their other energy source: the voice! Your forearms are energetically connected to your voice. So, while you're most likely engaging in repetitive movements that are putting extra stress on your forearms, if you're having trouble in this area, you must also ask yourself this: Is there something that you are not talking about? Are you feeling one way but just really haven't had the gumption to bring it up and discuss it thoroughly? Do you feel unheard, even if you do say how you are feeling? Is this striking a chord with you? Do you love to sing but won't sing in front of people? Even if you are a closet singer, are you allowing yourself little concerts often enough, say in your car? Strive to be open, creative, responsive, and willing to engage in your creative communications. Expressing yourself and giving heed to your own voice is a powerful key to healing the emotions stored in the forearms.

✖ THE FOREARMS SELF-RELEASE EXERCISE

Place the knuckles of each hand together with your elbows bent. Your fingertips and backs of the hands rest against each other with your fingertips facing down. Lower your elbows below the plane where the wrists are. If you are unable to lower the elbows below the line, this is a possible indicator of carpal tunnel issues in your forearm extensors. See a professional for help with this, and, in the meantime, continue to practice this stretch often, trying to bring the elbows down gently.

Seated Carpal Tunnel Stretch

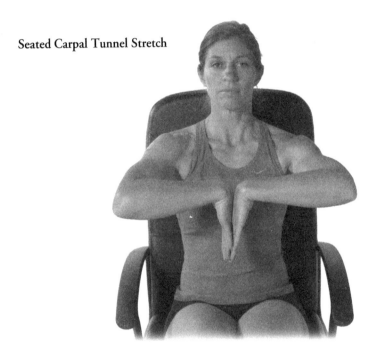

The Hands

The thenar and hypothenar are the largest muscle group of the hands. The thenar is the largest, and its purpose is to bring the thumb all the way across the hands. It can connect the pinky to the thumb. Thumbs are opposable and a large distinction between animals and humans. In the wrist (the retinaculum), there is nothing but tendons. The muscles exist in the palms and in the forearms. They do not exist in the wrists or in the fingers. Everything that pulls, grips, and spreads from the belly of those muscles is located in the forearms.

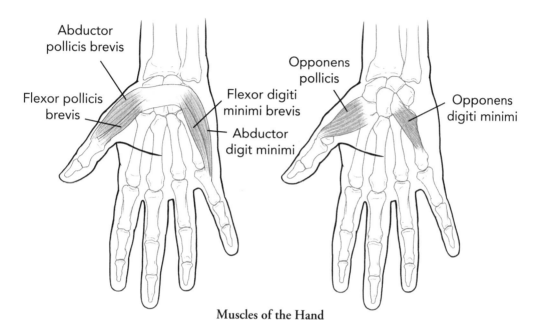

Abductor pollicis brevis

Flexor pollicis brevis

Opponens pollicis

Flexor digiti minimi brevis

Abductor digit minimi

Opponens digiti minimi

Muscles of the Hand

Thenar muscles are made up of flexor pollicis brevis, abductor pollicis brevis, and opponens pollicis. These make the thumbs move toward the fingers and away from the fingers.

The hypothenar muscles are made up of flexor digiti minimi brevis, abductor digiti minimi, and opponens digiti minimi. They move the pinky finger close to the other fingers and away from the other fingers.

There are deeper tiny muscles that assist the fingers in splaying or connecting motion. The muscles are located in the top of the hands and not in the fingers. The tendons in the fingers accomplish flexion and extension and are moved by the muscles in the forearms.

The hands are a spectacular part of the body to study because it both gives and receives so much information. Your hands tell your story. The hands are where the most energy is released in bodywork and where information is received through increasing the palpation skills. In the fingertips, there are more nerve endings than almost any other place in the entire body. The sensitivity in the fingers and hands can be incredible, especially if you work with it. If the energy is open, you will know it by two things: (1) the hands will become warm, and (2) you might be able to see splotchy white spots that appear in the palms of the hands and even on the skin over the fingers as energy is moving out of your hands. When I used to practice tai chi with my teacher, he always walked by and checked our hands for those two things to ensure that the chi was in fact moving and our channels were fully open. The hands also give and receive information based on the right side or the left. The right side is the giver and the left side is the receiver. This goes with energy, and it is the same when something happens to us, as we tend to store that pain or pressure on one side or the other depending.

Going even further, the lines on the palms of the hands tell your story, too. Your life line, head line, heart line, fate line, and more are located on the palms of your hands. The left hand is more about your soul map. These are things that you are slated with coming into this life. The right hand lines can change more so than the left side, depending on life experience. Basically, the left is what spirit gave you for this life and the right is what you've done with it.

Here is an example: A few years ago, a friend of mine lost her significant other. When it happened, the event showed up as a cross on the palm of her hand. She knew whether a palm reader was the real deal based on whether or not they noticed this cross and asked her about it. She would go to people who could look at the palm of her right hand (the hand that is more related to personal experience) and they would ask her "What happened to you in your twenties?" That question was solely based by a person reading the lines in her palms.

Your hands tell your story. When you prepare food, your hands touch the food and love or whatever thoughts you are thinking transfer into the food. When food is made with someone's love, we can feel it. All of our senses are intimately connected and our hands are a spectacular part of that mix. Energy transfers through the hands both in giving loving energy and taking in energy. If you were to cause physical harm to someone, it is likely done through the hands. Your hands can be used in the worst of ways and the greatest of ways. Think of your hands as sacred magic. Use them wisely.

Suggested Stones for the Arms and Shoulders

These stones will help support you in releasing any tensions held in the muscles of the arms. Their energies encourage you to be more open to allowing and embracing.

Aventurine: Opens us to new opportunities, again helping us to receive.

Quartz crystals: Helps us to clear the mind and not only set our intentions but also follow through with them from a higher perspective.

Rose quartz: The ideal stone for unconditional love. Be open to the most gentle, loving kindness that rose quartz can give to the wearer.

Turquoise: Is a master healing stone. Use this after you have done proper clearing work and get into a space that you feel worthy to receive the benefits of this wonder stone. You can wear it or keep it in your pocket or close by.

Suggested Essential Oils for the Arms and Shoulders

These oils will help you open to the energies of receiving as you work with the muscles of the arms.

Frankincense oil: Applied to pains in the arms, forearms, or shoulders is believed to help relieve the physical pain as well as help ground the emotions. Mix it with your favorite carrier oil to nourish your skin and soothe your soul. (Great carrier oils are grapeseed, jojoba, coconut, and olive.)

Neroli or Orange Blossom Oil: Known for its calming and healing effects on the mind, body, and spirit. Use this oil to connect you to your highest self as you clear away the feelings of being unworthy.

Rose oil: Correlates to the fourth chakra (this is the heart chakra, but it's also in line with the shoulders), helping to harmonize your entire being with loving energy. This oil will help you be open to receiving love in the purest form. Use this with a diffuser to invigorate your senses and promote calm, loving feelings.

⌘ Meditation for the Arms and Shoulders

Anything that deals with being able to receive directly correlates to feelings of being worthy. We block the ability to see ourselves as worthy of receiving certain gifts, especially gifts offered with nothing needed in return. This is all the arms and shoulders. Feeling worthy to receive is paramount for the arms and shoulders to change their tune to one of abundance and acceptance of loving kindness.

Breathe deeply into your own body. Breathe deeply into the space around you. Prepare your mind to claim your life in a stronger and more positive way through your breath and through intention. First start by breathing a little louder than you usually would. Really allow your exhales to be loud and come from a deeper place. This is a *take in and let go* breathing pattern.

Inhale one word that describes something that you want to bring into you. Exhale a word that describes something you are ready to let go of. Some examples are:

Inhale love	Exhale fear
Inhale peace	Exhale frustration
Inhale joy	Exhale sadness
Inhale vitality	Exhale confusion
Inhale healthy being	Exhale unwanted habits
Inhale truth	Exhale dissolution

Notice with the words coming in and out of your mind that you keep coming back to one set of affirmations. Continue to repeat the words that resonate the strongest within you for today. Close your eyes and breathe deeply into the belly and relax your heart and mind. Slowly let the words go and now just focus on the breath only coming in and going out. Continue this until you get to a still point and everything is calm and steady. Come out of this practice very slowly. Keep the words that you chose in your heart throughout the day or night.

Chapter 9

The Chest
Your Storehouse for
What's at the Heart of the Matter

The muscles of the chest keep the posture upright and work directly with the muscles in the upper and middle back. When one opens, the other closes and vice versa. We must remain at a balance of keeping both the chest and the back straight in good posture for both to remain open. The chest (along with the triceps) pushes weight or emotions away from the body as well as brings weight or energy toward the body (with the biceps).

The pectoralis major fans the entire chest from the breastbone to the shoulder. Underneath the pec major is the pectoralis minor. The movement in the chest is to create movement in the arms. It also helps with inhalation, pulling the ribs up so that the lungs can expand fully. Pec minor works with the serratus anterior to create full range of movement for the scapula. It originates from three ribs (third, fourth, and fifth) and inserts to the coracoid process of the scapula. Together these muscles move the arms.

The chest is primarily thought of as the house of the heart chakra. The emotions associated with this area are love, hate, and sadness. The lungs govern sadness while the heart space covers love and/or hate. The chest as a whole is associated with the nurturing spirit. Embracing life, love, acceptance, and kindness, or opposite to this—feeling unloved, not accepted, unappreciated, repelled, angry, hateful, or sad—are all emotions that will show in the chest. When we see the shoulders rolling forward, it brings the chest farther away from receiving love from the outside. The heart chakra/chest area goes into hiding.

When we are in a really good positive place, we stand up straighter, opening our chest and our hearts to new and loving experiences.

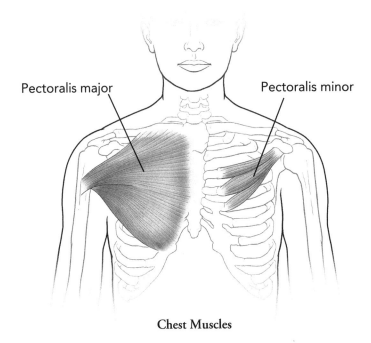

Pectoralis major

Pectoralis minor

Chest Muscles

This area in the body is a sensitive area physically as well as energetically, and we must treat it with care. When practicing energy work, I bring my open hands to the center of the chest and hold them in this space for at least three minutes. If a person is not willing to let you in, feel free to place one hand on the front of the chest (above the breasts) and the other hand underneath the body in the same location. The front is much more guarded than coming into the chest from the backside. I allow the person to feel the effects of loving kindness with absolutely no ulterior motives. I know they are releasing if I hear the deep sigh of relief that happens when they allow the healing energy to enter. You may very well get a full release from working in this space—tears, coughing, sneezing, sadness, gladness, acceptance, tolerance, joy…one never knows ahead of time how an emotional release will manifest. The chest muscles surround the treasure of the soul and the sacred heart space.

❀ THE CHEST SELF-RELEASE EXERCISE

There are two self-release exercises that work with the chest. I'll describe each below with an additional modification for the second.

The Prayer Pose

Bringing the energy into the heart space is easy to do when you place your palms together at the heart chakra. It's why we use it in prayers, contemplation, yoga, meditation, and gratitude giving. Bringing the energy of the palms and uniting it with the energy of the heart is powerful. Practice this often to center and clear your mind and align it with your heart. This is the time to repeat the magic words: *Thank you. Thank you. Thank you.* Give yourself love, kindness, and a million thanks for the spectacular person that you are and the love that you are receiving in this space.

Prayer Pose

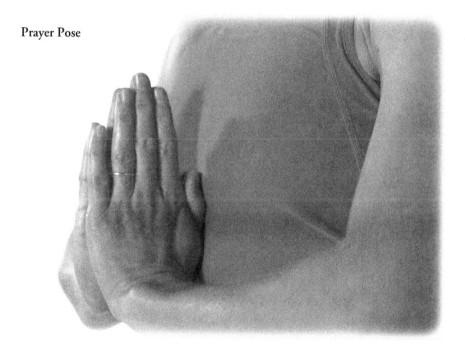

The Reverse Prayer Stretch

This is a stretch to open the muscles of the chest. It comes easily to some body types and less so for others. To do the reverse prayer stretch, place your hands behind your back and connect your pinky fingers first against each other. This will anchor you to direct all the other fingertips and thumbs to face upward as you then press the hands together for support. If you are able to do this pose, be sure to keep your chin up so that the heart center and chest muscles can fully open.

If you are unable to do flat palms to each other, simply grabbing your elbows behind your back is also wonderful for self-release. Clasping the hands and straightening the arms behind your back is also a great chest opener if the other two aren't comfortable for you to do.

Reverse Prayer Pose

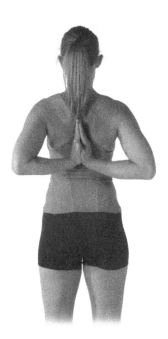

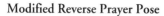

Modified Reverse Prayer Pose

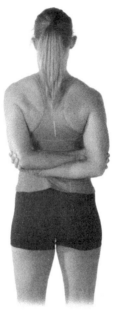

Affirmations

When you engage in the self-release exercise, you are targeting the specific muscle group. Adding in the affirmation at the same time connects the body with the mind and strengthens your intentions for the highest outcome. For every affirmation, choose one or more statement that best fits where you are currently or create your own. Repeat the statement throughout the day.

- I am *love*.
- I am an all-encompassing being of pure love and joy.
- I radiate kindness and compassion for myself and others.
- I am open to receiving and giving love without attachment.
- I choose love as my primary emotion.

Suggested Stones for the Chest

The power of stones can also be utilized to help balance and heal your chest and the heart chakra these muscles protect.

Green aventurine: A sacred healing stone for the heart. This stone provides love and support to the wearer.

Green calcite: A wonderful healing stone for the heart center/chest. A subtle stone that encourages healing and openness.

Rose quartz: The top stone for such endeavors. This is a stone of unconditional love and it can be worn by absolutely any person. The rose quartz is used in the process of soul retrieval. In exchange for recovering your soul pieces, a piece of rose quartz is given in its place to bring your soul pieces back to you to make you whole again. No stone is as sweet and as pure as the beloved rose quartz.

Turquoise: A versatile and powerful stone that is also good for love and healing because it is such a powerful stone. This is a great stone to wear over the chest for healing physically, spiritually, and emotionally.

Suggested Essential Oils for the Chest

These essential oils are also beneficial in working with the emotions of the chest:

Lavender: Is always a loving oil that promotes kind, gentle healing and compassion. You really can't go wrong with using lavender for any form of healing through oils. You can apply lavender oil directly to the skin. I like to use it on my temples and the center of my chest to promote sacred, gentle healing.

Neroli: Has a vibrational frequency that aids in opening the heart chakra, harmonizing the mind and emotions while uplifting the spirit. This oil encourages confidence, joy, and peace.

Rose oil: It is believed to have the highest spiritual frequency of all the oils. This opens the heart, clearing the way for unconditional love. Think of rose oil as the oil version of the rose quartz stone.

⌘ Meditation for the Chest

I collaborated with clinical hypnotherapist Shaye Hudson, MA, LPC, C.Ht for this particular meditation. Not many people can assist in going down deep into our heart spaces the way a hypnotherapist is able to. Practice this meditation often:

More and more people in the world crave hope. We all need some hope that things will get better when we find ourselves in spaces that we are unsure of or when we have experienced loss. It is cliché to say that love begins from within, but there is no truer truth in all reality. It must begin from within. You must learn to fall in love with yourself and cultivate a love that is so liberating that you have it radiating from down deep no matter where you are. This meditation will help restore hope and promote feelings of healing, nurturing, and self-love. If you have a rose quartz, now is the time to place it on your chest. If not, then just place your own hands over your heart. Lie down and get comfortable. Close your eyes and begin to search through your hands or with your stone down deep into your heart space.

Place your attention on your breath. Notice that when you are breathing in through your nose the air is cool and when you are breathing out through your mouth the air is warm. Breathe normally. Let's now fill your body with the cool crisp air from mother nature's life-giving energy. Take a deep breath in through your nose. All the way in. Filling your abdomen. Now exhale completely all the way to the bottom of your lungs. All the way out. Do it again. All the way in. Now exhaling all the way out. One more time and this time when you have filled your lungs with clean, calming, and relaxing energy hold it in for moment. Now let it out slowly and allow yourself to relax more deeply. Allow your mind to go deeper and deeper into the heart space within.

Now imagine a wave of relaxing energy beginning from the top of your head, flowing down your face, relaxing the space behind your eyes. Relaxing your cheeks, your jaw, with the teeth not quite touching. Relaxing your neck, shoulders, chest, and upper back. Relaxing your waist and lower back. Relaxing your hips, thighs, knees, calves, feet, and toes, running into the ground. Feeling deeper, grounded, and relaxed.

Place your attention into your heart center. Imagine the faces of those who you love and care about. It could be family members, friends, or pets. See their faces one by one and notice what you love and appreciate about them. It could be a way they smile, act, sound, look, or a touching moment when you were with them. Now allow the love and appreciation in your heart space to well up. See their faces one by one and send each one your love. Imagine this love as a brilliant, healing, nurturing light flowing from your heart center directly to theirs. Take the next few moments to feel this love, let it intensify, and send this energy to each person from your heart space.

Imagine now receiving their love from those you just imagined into your heart. See their faces one by one pouring this light of love into your heart center. Feel this loving, warm, and nurturing energy welling up and intensifying. Imagine this brilliant light flowing into your heart center and the crystal. Take the next few moments to receive and feel this loving, nurturing, and warm energy. Feel it move and expand deeply into your heart. See it healing, clearing, and filling your heart space. Be willing to accept such love as deeply and as unselfishly as you directed it to them.

Now focus on your rose quartz crystal. See your crystal grow in brilliance until the entire room is filled with light. This is your light. See this light all around you. Shining on you. Feel this energy in this light. It feels healing, nurturing, and full of self-love. Let this light flow throughout your body now, filling your heart space completely. Pushing away all fears. Clearing away all doubts. You are now filled with this light. You are powerful and radiant glowing with the shining light from your own heart.

Take the next few moments to rest into the being of your own healing, nurturing, and loving light. Embrace and experience yourself as the absolutely divine, radiant, loving being that you are. When you are ready to come back to the room and to your conscious awareness count up from ten to one. When you reach one, you will be awake, alert, feeling centered in the heart, and back to your full awareness.

Chapter 10

The Head, Face, and Jaws
Your Storehouse for
Gaining Clarity and a Wider Vision

The head, face, jaws, and neck are associated with flexibility and rigidity and with the ability to see with clarity and wider vision. These areas are the emotional storehouse of energies associated with seeing things in a clear perspective.

Anatomy Overview of the Muscles of Facial Expression

Frontalis: Moves the muscles in the forehead.

Orbicularis oculi: Moves the muscles around the eyes. Closes eyes and squints.

Orbicularis oris: Moves the muscles around the mouth. Pursing the lips, closing the lips.

Zygomatic muscle: Is the smile muscle.

Buccinator: Brings the cheeks in toward the teeth.

Levator labii superioris: Elevates the upper lip.

Depressor labii inferioris: Depresses the lower lip.

Nasalis: Opens and closes your nostrils.

Mentalis: The two muscles that make up the chin and are affected when you cry or pout.

An exercise for relaxing this area is to place your cupped palms over your eyes. Notice that the base of your hands rest on the zygomatic arch, or the cheekbones. With the palms of the hands, slightly pull outward to open the nostrils and relax the cheeks. With the cupped palms directly over the eyes, send through your palms healing energy to the eyes. The eyes can get so tired and we want to send them loving, warm, healing thoughts, even envisioning flowers coming through your hands into the eyes, an offering of love and warmth. If you love daisies, envision beautiful white or yellow daisies on the insides of your palms coming through and into the eyes. Project whatever image onto your palms that can give your eyes the offering of positivity and light.

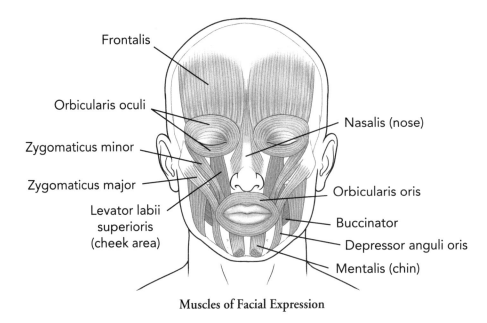

Muscles of Facial Expression

When we think of the temple, we just think of the soft spot outside of the corner of the eyes, but the muscle actually spans along the entire ear and side of the head. Massaging with your fingers not just in that soft area but all the way around your ears and head to the base of the skull is a great stress reliever. The head itself is covered with fascia. It holds a lot of tension and can easily relax with simple massage techniques. As crazy as this sounds, by gently grabbing as much hair as you are able to and gently pulling up helps to relieve the fascia in the head, bringing quickly to you some real *Ahhhh* moments! Gather up the hair, gently pull it up, and then release and gather up another area of hair and repeat until all of the hair on the head has been gently gathered and released.

The Jaws

The muscles of the head and face are primarily used for moving the mandible when we speak or chew, as the mandible is the only freely movable bone in the human skull. The main muscles involved in mastication are the lateral pterygoid (opens the jaw and protrudes the mandible sideward), the masseter muscle, the medial pterygoid, and the temporalis (all three close the jaw and clench the teeth).

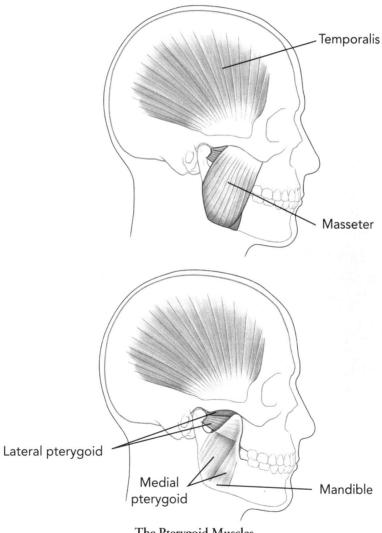

The Pterygoid Muscles

Emotionally, we all chew on the stresses of life, as well as chewing on food (our sustenance). The jaws store deep tensions. Miscommunications that so often take place now that we use so much technology to communicate can manifest as emotional stress and physical tension that hangs deep into the jaws. Any text or e-mail can set us off, and we clench our jaws and begin a strong mental cycle based off a total miscommunication. The same reaction occurs if the communication was perfectly understood but painful to hear.

The high emotional component of the jaws is the idea behind the expression "chewing on the bone." When you play a conversation over and over again in your head, the aches and pains of the hurt you feel most often go to bed deep into the jaw muscles. They tuck themselves in and prepare for a long winter's nap in this area. If you are the type of person who thinks about something, then thinks about it some more, and then more with an analysis of whatever you are thinking about, and again some more, you might be someone with jaw problems. Too many times, this area gets looked over when releasing the body from stress. Honestly, it should be one of the first places to check.

The jaws and the neck go hand in hand. If your neck is tight and you are experiencing tension headaches often, treating the jaws can unlock and release all of those areas. The jaws are a storage space for old pains, anguish, shame, and anger. It is your storage space for things said and not said that were hurtful.

If you can see a professional massage therapist who has completed intraoral training, it can be a true game changer. Having someone go inside the mouth and treat the pterygoid muscles and the masseter can relieve you of unimaginable stress. If you have never had this work, please go in search of someone who knows how to manually release those muscles for you.

❀ The Jaw Self-Release Exercise

The lateral (and medial) pterygoid muscles are hidden inside the mouth, but if you line up your three fingers just under the zygomatic arch (the cheekbone) and open your mouth, you will notice just under your middle finger that there is something that pops up. That is the lateral pterygoid and that muscle is a very important one. You can take your middle finger and massage side to side over this notch to help release the pain in this area.

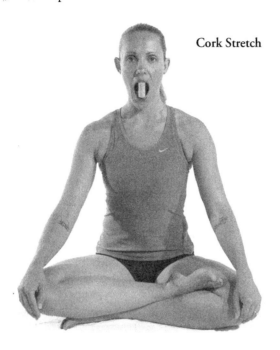

Cork Stretch

Another great jaw release that I am a huge fan of using is a cork stretch (like the cork from a wine bottle or you can get them by the bagful at any craft store). Hold the cork vertically between the top and bottom teeth. Hold it in place for a minimum of three minutes for best results. You will drool. It's okay. This will release all of the jaw muscles and the muscles that fan around the whole temporalis. I keep a cork in my glove compartment and pull it out when I find that I am stressed out or clenching my teeth—which usually occurs when I'm stuck in traffic! I have many clients that also keep corks on hand, and they use them often with great results. I think this is one of those sage pieces of wisdom that isn't shared nearly enough.

❀ THE EYEBROWS SELF-RELEASE EXERCISE

The muscles in the eyebrows can hold a lot of negative energy. This is probably due to the wrinkling of the eyebrows, squinting the eyes, and squeezing the middle of the eyebrows together when you are angry. In Chinese medicine, they call the lines to the inside of the eyebrows to be the liver/gallbladder lines of anger. If you were to go to a plastic surgeon, they would call these lines the elevens. This is the desired area to get Botox if you're into that kind of thing.

Eyebrow Stretch—Part 1

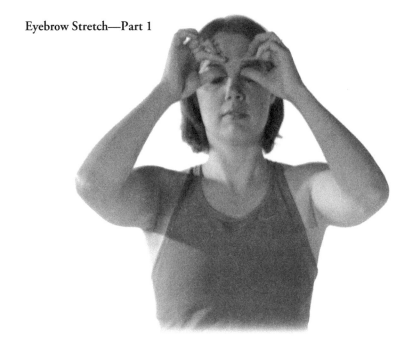

Eyebrow Stretch—Part 2

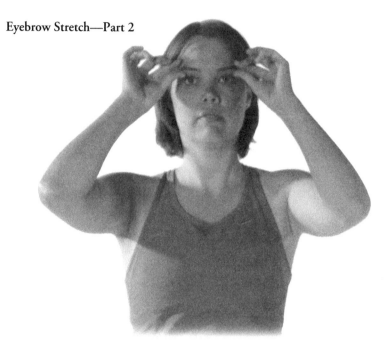

To release that pent-up energy, simply pinch your eyebrows from the very inside toward the eye first, using both hands at the same time with one on each of your eyebrows. Pinch and hold, then to the middle of the eyebrow, pinch and hold, and to the outside corners of the eyebrow, pinch and hold. Repeat this at least three times through.

Affirmations

When you engage in the self-release exercise, you are targeting the specific muscle group. Adding in the affirmation at the same time connects the body with the mind and strengthens your intentions for the highest outcome. For every affirmation, choose one or more statement that best fits where you are currently or create your own. Repeat the statement throughout the day.

- I *express*.
- I allow myself to be honest and forthcoming with information.
- I do not hold back my own feelings or emotions.
- I do not speak harshly, but I do speak truthfully.
- I acknowledge that the muscles of facial expression reveal my feelings.
- I allow myself to feel freedom throughout my entire being.
- I no longer hang on to things and chew on the bone that no longer serves me.

❋ Self-Release Stretch for All Muscles of Facial Expression

This exercise is called the lion. Begin by inhaling and holding your breath. At the same time, close your eyes tight and clench your jaws tight. Then with a loud, roaring exhale open your eyes wide and stick out your tongue as far as you can. Open up the muscles of facial expression and give that deep roaring energy to the exhale. Do this a few times over.

Next, make it more interesting. Keep doing the breathing patterns and the facial expressions of the lion but now go deeper. Inhale and take in a word that will help you to realize what you are feeling. Exhale and say a word of emotion that must be let out. Example: inhale *Warrior* and think that you are a warrior right now, hunting out your own demons. Exhale and say *Gotcha!* and release whatever feeling, words, or energies that have been hiding down deep. Keep changing up your words for both inhale and exhale. You could do things like inhale *stillness* and exhale *anger*. They're your words to play with and your feelings to find and release. Play like a lion but mean business as you work this.

Suggested Stones for the Mouth and Face

Amber: A useful stone for teeth, helping to ease pains in the gums and mouth.

Clear quartz: A great stone that can be used to purify the energy in this area. This is a wonderful stone to place over the third eye to help you calm the face, strengthen your intention, and raise your frequency.

Lemurian crystals: Thought to be stones from Atlantis containing etched bar codes of information to help guide us in the present times. Use this stone to help balance your yin energy or to help you attune to a higher vibration of clarity to embrace a new level of spiritual enlightenment. This activates the high crown chakra and connects your energies to the ether. It is a wonderful stone to put at the third eye or at the top of the head.

Selenite: Can be used to attune the whole body and face to a higher vibration. This stone helps to raise and harness the power of intention, as it provides its own healing energies.

Smokey quartz: Helps to clear away any negative energy. Use this to place on your face during meditations or wear it as a necklace. This stone is a great stone for clearing and healing.

Sodalite: A great stone for the head, helping to open the third eye and also ease sinus issues. It can be utilized in TMJ and to aid in visualization and manifesting your goals.

Sugilite: This is the stone that calls forth the Archangel Michael. It is a powerful stone of a dark purple with reddish and blue hues. This is a stone to place high on the face or third eye or higher. It is a wonderful necklace to have as well.

Suggested Essential Oils for the Mouth and Face

Amber oil: Can be used in a diffuser or diluted with a carrier oil to help relieve pain in the jaws and teeth or to help dispel any negative energy you may have attracted. Burning amber oil helps to clear your own personal body space.

Cedarwood: Can be used in a diffuser to ground your energies and call forth a deep sleep. This oil can help you relax the entire face so that you hold no tensions as you drift off into dreamland.

Lavender: Is always a great oil to be able to apply directly to the skin. Use at the temples or at the third eye for a calming, relaxing effect. Lavender also has a natural antibiotic property to it. It can be used on young people up to geriatric. This is a very safe and loving oil to use.

Ylang Ylang: Can be used to invoke happiness, calm, and ease. The face holds so much emotional tension, we want to encourage happiness to release the frown lines and calm the muscles that reveal our worries. This can be put directly on the skin or with a carrier oil or placed in a diffuser. I personally like to put this oil in my navel and on my third eye and top of my head for a feeling of calm and centered joy.

✖ MEDITATION FOR THE MOUTH AND FACE

Too often anything that has happened to us in our lives has rested deeply within our jaws as we continue to replay the scenario over and over again each time with a different way we wish we might have responded or handled it. The replay becomes so deeply entrenched within our beings that not only do we chew on it, but our face begins to show signs that there is something that we just can't seem to let go of. Lines show up in certain areas of our faces based on our emotions. Our secret hideaway of replay then becomes something that shines outward for others to glimpse of us as well. There comes a point where we have to let go of the past and stop replaying the pains like a song stuck right in that place that stays on repeat. It's time to fast forward to the next song of our life's experiences and leave this song behind.

Open your eyes and look at the situation one last time. Take it all in. Be with it and sit with it and feel every inch of the memory that you hold so dear to you even though with it is all unpleasant sensations that set off up and down your being. Go into it. Open your hands and your arms. Open your eyes and your body. Sit in a space with your arms out, fingers spread, legs out, feet open, eyes open, forehead lines raised, even your mouth can be open. Take it all in. Think about it for one full final time so that when I ask you to put it away, there won't be pieces left for you to chase after and pick up again. Feel the feelings. Replay things said and things done. Replay the part you played; replay the part anyone else played. Feel your feelings and be totally open and honest about your feelings in this space.

Now lie down and close your eyes. Extend your arms and legs, open your hands, and relax your feet. Let it wash over you, but this time don't keep it. Still lying on your back, feel all of those feelings that you just opened up to begin at the top of your head and now melt like a pat of butter on top of your head, on the tops of your shoulders, over your face, over your chest, past your ears, down your arms and your hands, and off your fingers. Off your middle body, down your legs, and off your feet. From any and every angle of your body let the melted butter of sorrow and anger leave your body. Drip by drip let it go off of every part of you. Breathe into this space and feel the warmth of the butter and the warmth of the old anger and resentment go with it. Dripping off your whole being. Let it melt and wash away.

Once it is off you, lay there as long as you can and notice how you feel in that moment, allowing that situation to finally melt down and off you. Feel the freed up space that is now in your mind and in your body. Feel the eyes soften and the stress you keep around your eyes release and all of a sudden no furrowed brow, no squinty eyes. Your nose softens and breath is easier to get in and out. Your ears relax. Your jaws relax and your top and bottom teeth don't touch. Your tongue softens and rests with ease down at the bottom of the mouth. Under the jaws into the front of the neck where the crease of the neck softens. Your heart opens up. Your body relaxes and you smile. Feel the feeling of the release. Embrace this feeling of release. It is yours to keep!

Stay in this space and breathe deeply, calmly, and openly into your whole body. Feel the face feel more beautiful and let the light of your soul shine up and out through your eyes and third eye. Allow the energy into your eyes and third eye from the heavens above. Interchange the energy and feel that all of a sudden the energy you are exchanging is of a much higher level. Be open to this new energy and let it lead the way. Go toward it in your mind and let it deep into your being. You are allowed to be happy. You are allowed to be free from pain. You are allowed to be free. You are allowed. You are. I am. We are. Peace it is. We are free.

Chapter 11

The Neck

Your Storehouse for Stress, Flexibility, Awareness, and Claiming Your Life

The basic physical overview of the entire neck can allow you to know many things. If you're not sleeping well, or you're not using good pillows, it will show in the muscles of the neck. If you are under tremendous stress or tension, if you clench your jaws or grind your teeth, if you're someone who just does not let go in any sense of the word—these issues will all reveal themselves as stress and tension in the muscles of the neck. The phrase "You are a pain in the neck!" comes from the emotional pains that can store themselves in the neck. Stress, pain, tension, and irritation all live in the neck. On the flip side, flexibility, awareness, and claiming your life can also be the opportunity from the neck area.

Sometimes the front of the neck will have issues due to a blockage of the throat chakra. This can happen if there is something you need to express or something that you have to say that needs to be heard. This area can also hold the emotional memory of trauma, such as being choked. The throat in particular is extremely delicate, but it is possible to treat this area to help release very old, very deep wounds or to help relieve the physical discomfort caused by a hoarse voice, whiplash, or other complaints. The neck is a magical and stress-filled part of the body for certain.

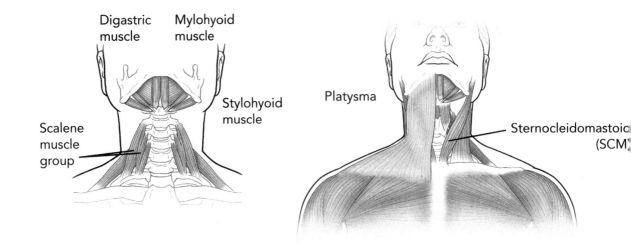

The Neck Front View

The neck represents your ability to be flexible. Do you look at situations with objectivity? Are you able to see more than one side of a situation? Do you give yourself the freedom to explore life beyond the scope of what other people expect from you? Do you honor your sacred path? Do you look deep within? Do you look deep outside of yourself? Your neck controls all of these things.

The neck represents quite a few things, including sight, sound, speech, smell, and taste. When the neck is tight either physically or emotionally, the vision is more narrow. People with tight necks and minimal flexibility in their neck may well be someone with limited flexibility in their general views as well. When we experience issues in the neck, there is a whole host of questions to be asked so we can get to the most accurate answers:

Is there something I'm not seeing?

Is there something that I want to say but feel I am not being heard or lack the strength and courage to say out loud?

How am I dealing with stress and what part do I play in any drama affecting my life?

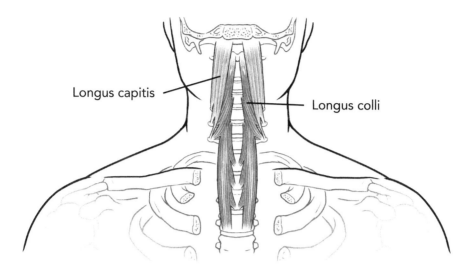

Deep Anterior Neck Muscles

The muscles to focus on at the front of the neck are the longus capitis, longus colli, and the sternocleidomastoid (SCM). There are several more muscles, but these cover the primary muscles of the anterior physical neck that will be our focus here. As we discuss the longus colli, we must realize that there is a physical treatment to this emotionally supercharged muscle. However, unless you have learned this from teachers or trained professionals, never attempt to treat this muscle. It is the most emotional muscle of the entire body. The longus colli holds trauma of all kinds. Physical trauma, such as being choked, strangled, or any violent act, sits within this muscle. It also holds more subtle trauma, such as things that you have not said, wish you had not said, being verbally abused. Not knowing what to do or sticking up for yourself or leaving the situation sits deeply within this area.

This is also the area that the throat chakra governs, so both physically and energetically this area holds on to the pain. Coughing with intention is the best release physically for this muscle. Even better for the emotional part is coughing followed by crying. This is the area that you can highly encourage serious body release. All the sadness, shame, guilt, fear, abuse, and pain leaves as you release from this muscle.

It is my belief that the foundation of the majority of emotional body issues stem from a disconnect in communication. Whether that be communication within your own body and confusing messages from within, painful communication, stifled communication with anyone in your life, or not saying what you really think and feel, all of this matters. If you are a person who finds themselves being incredibly mean and spiteful when you are angry and saying things just for the purpose of causing pain, understand that it doubles within yourself and holds on tight in this muscle area. No ill will goes unpunished. If you are someone who uses words to cause harm, stop it right now. Change your direction and your method of communication. This healing starts from within and you must make the changes to your behaviors if you are ever to bring full healing to your whole being. If you are the opposite and hold everything in for fear of ever hurting anyone's feelings, you too have some work to do. Communication is the foundation of hurt and the key to releasing it. If you have been in an abusive situation, think about the way that someone spoke to you. If anyone has mishandled you by way of threatening language, your body will forever feel that pain unless you can find your way through it to detach yourself from those words.

People can be very mean and words hurt down to the bones. For the sake of your longus colli and your ultimate healing, go back to your past and visit the times where someone caused you great pains through their words and work with yourself to remove them to the point that you no longer identify with that pain. Look to your future and be sure to clear your own patterns of communication. Learn to be assertive, not vicious. Learn to speak up and to honor who you are and where you are in any given process. Take control over your life and own your own part as you play the various roles to others. Now is the time to own your sh*t. *Own it.* Come into it. Get deep with self-awareness, figure out who you are, and own it. Get clean. Run your life from a clean workspace within. Think of a water faucet. Match the intensity of how much water comes out with whatever you are experiencing currently in your emotional space. Then as you visualize the water being very clean, clear, and crisp, identify yourself with that water in how you behave in your life. Repeat: "I run clean." Come from that space with how you speak to yourself and others.

I used to have a deeper and more raspy voice. I always assumed it was because of the years of cheerleading that I put my yelling voice through. The first time I had my longus colli released, my voice actually changed. It is now the voice that it used to be from years before many traumas occurred. I wish I could explain this part better to you, but it is something that you might need to experience for yourself. My voice was restored through this work. This is different from a friend who had whiplash after a car accident and was left without a voice. I did this work and her voice returned at least 50 percent the same day as the accident. That is physical. That was purely a physical release from the trauma of the neck being forced in a forward direction opposite of the natural curvature of the spine. Whiplash is one thing, and physically releasing the muscle of the longus colli requires a shift of the trachea to be able to treat the spine of the neck from the front side. The restoring of my voice was something that was given back to me and helped me to reunite with a part of myself. It was a profound experience to get up off the table and hear a different voice coming out of me. It was perfect. I will forever be grateful that releasing these muscles in the front of my neck allowed me to heal and restore a part of myself that I didn't even understand was missing until that moment.

The sternocleidomastoid (SCM) is a major muscle of note as well, and we will all recognize this muscle once you see it. It starts at the corner of the clavicle (collarbone) and connects just behind the jaw. This muscle is used all the time. If you have a cough, this muscle will be very sore. If you lift weights, this muscle will be very sore. This muscle is strong and aids in turning the head from side to side. It is what is called an ipsilateral muscle, meaning that the muscle on the side you are turning toward is the muscle that is flexing. So the right side SCM turns the head to the right side, not the opposite side the way some other muscles do.

Energetically, the SCM muscle is a doozy. It is the chewer, the stabilizer, and the aggressor. It aids in whatever emotion you are experiencing. If you are angry and you yell, this muscle is a big part of it. If you are chewing on something and not able to let it go, this muscle is part of it. If you are building strength both internally and externally, this muscle is a big player. If there is pressure applied to this muscle (sifting is what we do to this muscle by pinching it from both sides and holding and sifting each part, starting from the bottom by the collarbones and repeating up to the top behind the jaws), the pain can radiate over the entire head and land inside the corner of the eyes.

This muscle truly is a powerhouse muscle. My teachers used to tell us not to let anyone off your table without treating the SCM. For both physical and emotional reasons, I agree completely on this sentiment. When looking at photos of strength lifters, you can recognize easily this muscle. They look like a V shaped muscle at the front of the neck. If you turn your own head to the side you can feel this muscle present itself. If you turn your head to the side and place your thumb on the inside line of this muscle and then bring your head back to center you can hold the other side of the muscle with the other fingers and hold the muscle between your thumb and fingers and give it a little squeeze. Feel the pressure and then the release. You can repeat this yourself, turning your head and getting a good hold on the muscle and working your way up, squeezing this muscle to help it soften. Don't get overly aggressive with it, and if you feel a pulse get off. This is a move that I do teach clients because this muscle is so important to keep healthy and flexible.

❁ THE ANTERIOR NECK (AND THE CHEST) SELF-RELEASE EXERCISE

This exercise is called the fish pose. Lying on your back, bring your hands underneath you as straight as you can get them. Bring your palms facing down to the ground underneath your buttocks. The legs are stretched out straight. Now sit up on your forearms and place the crown of your head to the ground behind you. The trick in this stretch is keeping your lips together. Do not keep your teeth together, but keep the lips touching each other. Feel your jaws and the entire front of the neck completely release. Place the tip of your tongue against the roof of the mouth while doing this. Breathe slow, deep breaths through the nose. To come out of the pose, gently lift the head and then lay back down. Then remove the arms to the sides. This stretch stimulates the parathyroid.

Fish Pose

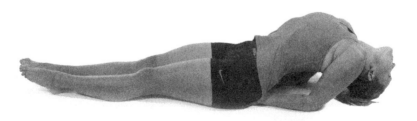

Affirmations

When you engage in the self-release exercise, you are targeting the specific muscle group. Adding in the affirmation at the same time connects the body with the mind and strengthens your intentions for the highest outcome. For every affirmation, choose one or more statement that best fits where you are currently or create your own. Repeat the statement throughout the day.

- I *synthesize*.
- I am willful in the most glorious way.
- I see the good in life.
- I chew and swallow with accuracy any situation life throws at me.
- I commit to seeing the whole picture.

Lateral Neck Muscles

When looking at the neck from the side, we want to be aware that the trapezius muscle group runs along this area, as well as the scalene muscles (anterior, middle, and posterior), still the SCM muscles, and platysma (the platysma is a superficial sheet of muscles that covers the muscles of the neck starting from the chest and shoulders). The scalene muscles aid in inspiration both physically as well as emotionally by lifting the ribs and helping you to be able to get a deeper breath in. Again, there are more muscles, but these are the big dogs of this area. It is in these muscles that turns the head.

The traps run from the top of the back of the neck, down the side of the neck, and then down to the upper mid back. It is in the traps and lower muscles around the shoulder blades that hold that knife in your back of betrayal. The scalenes connect into this emotional component because it is here that we are able to move our head and our eyes to see what is going on around us. When this muscle is locked down, or we are blind to the situations before they hurt us, it is in this area that the pre-war pains are stored. What could I have done? Why didn't I know this was coming? What didn't I see? This is all in those lateral muscles of the neck. This is your awareness into the backside of your energy body. If these muscles are not open, neither is your full range of vision. These muscles need to be massaged, stretched, and spoken to in a loving way.

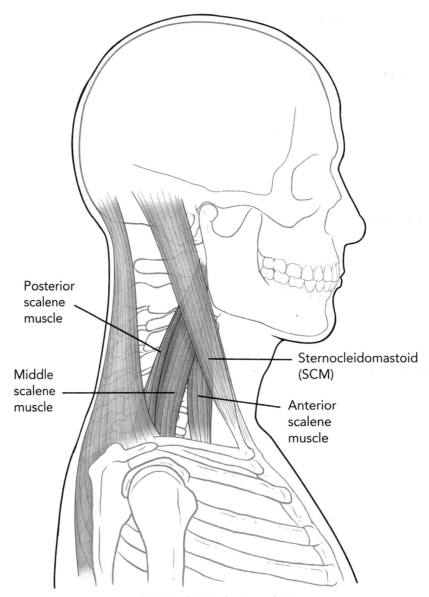

Posterior scalene muscle

Sternocleidomastoid (SCM)

Middle scalene muscle

Anterior scalene muscle

The Neck Muscles Lateral View

Acknowledging that these muscles hold the key is important. In the movie *My Big Fat Greek Wedding,* the mother made a great statement: "Yes, the man is the head of the house, but the woman is the neck. And she can turn the head any way she wants." That is very true in all aspects physically, emotionally, as well as energetically. As a therapist, I treat this area of the neck with the client in side lying posture. If you are a therapist or bodyworker and you don't currently treat the neck from this position, I highly encourage you to add that to your toolbox.

❀ THE LATERAL NECK SELF-RELEASE EXERCISE

Simple neck stretches are easy to do. However, more times than not, the simple neck stretches end up not being executed properly; therefore, you don't end up getting as good of a stretch as you really need to have. When we just stretch our necks to the side and bring the ear toward the shoulder, without realizing it's happening, we often lift our shoulder to meet the ear instead. To ensure that we keep the shoulders down and get a proper full neck stretch that engages all of the muscles on the side of the neck and the platysma, I have added in some extra steps.

Lateral Neck Stretch

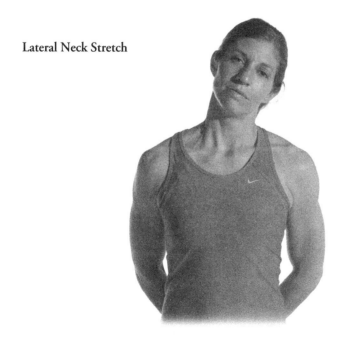

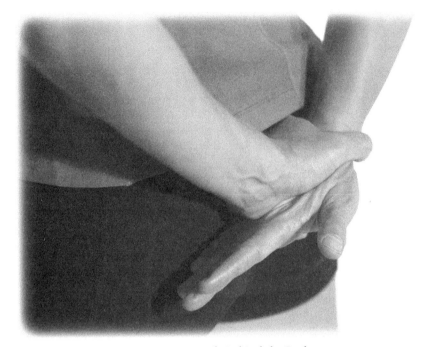

Hands Behind the Back

Begin by placing your hands behind your back. To stretch the right side, hold your right wrist with your left hand and gently bring your left ear toward the left shoulder. We hold the hands behind the back so that you will not be able to lift the shoulder up to meet the ear. Try to bring the hands down as low as you are able at the same time as stretching the neck. Open the mouth until you feel the stretch all the way up the side into the ear itself. Change sides and repeat.

Affirmations

When you engage in the self-release exercise, you are targeting the specific muscle group. Adding in the affirmation at the same time connects the body with the mind and strengthens your intentions for the highest outcome. For every affirmation, choose one or more statement that best fits where you are currently or create your own. Repeat the statement throughout the day.

- I am *flexible*.
- I can see life clearly.
- I do not bury my head in the sand.
- I see the world around me in all its glories and its messes.

Posterior Neck

This area of the body is what I think of as the mother ship. Starting just at the base of the head and top of the neck there is an area called the occipital ridge. It is the bones of the head and the muscles and fasciae just below this area. This is the money spot in my opinion. So much releases in this area. Just to the sides of the spine (the atlas to be more precise) immediately off the vertebra, correlates through to the eyes. One finger over from that, it correlates to the jaws. This is the backdoor release areas to the jaws and face. If the neck can't relax, we treat the jaws. If the jaws can't relax, we treat the base of the skull. These muscles go hand in hand in a huge way.

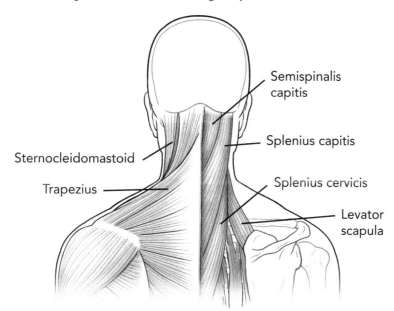

The Neck Muscles Rear View

Sadly, nowadays many states have banned intraoral work for reasons completely lost to me. I find the intraoral work to be absolutely of the utmost importance if I am going to get to those deep areas in their posterior (backside) of the neck to give it up. When they relax into this position, you will soon hear a great big breath in and out. In that moment, you free them from all the internal dialogue and stress that usually happens. The muscles to know in the back of the neck are semispinalis capitis, splenius capitis, and longissimus. Also the trapezius runs on top of them all. The other one to know is levator scapula which starts at the base of the skull and inserts into the top corner of the scapula (the top back of the shoulder blade).

Emotionally I don't want to let you in too deep! This is also precisely the location of having someone be a pain in your neck. We carry a whole host of tension from outside circumstances in this area. The posterior neck holds on to the same issues that the jaws do, the same issues that the traps do, the same issues that the shoulders do—it all connects into that area of the neck. The back of the neck holds the majority of tension in the body because it takes on so many emotions from all of their related spaces. Even financial worry lives in this area! Not only does that live in the low back but it also finds space to rent in the neck. This area of the body is stronger than the anterior neck so it has a little bit more energy and physical protection. I like to think of it, however, not so much as protection as a meaty muscle that doesn't let you in nearly as easily.

⌘ The Posterior Neck Self-Release Exercise

To release this muscle, the movement is a simple nodding of the head, bringing the chin down to the chest and up to the ceiling. There are also tools on the market for you to rest your head on that apply pressure to the base of the skull, accessing the occiput. They can be referred to as still point releases. You can create a makeshift still point release with two tennis balls by placing the balls just at the top of the neck beneath the ridge of the skull. Gently move your head side to side and work the tense areas in this part of your neck. Move slowly and with great intention and do not rub on the spine itself.

Affirmations

When you engage in the self-release exercise, you are targeting the specific muscle group. Adding in the affirmation at the same time connects the body with the mind and strengthens your intentions for the highest outcome. For every affirmation, choose one or more statement that best fits where you are currently or create your own. Repeat the statement throughout the day.

- I *trust*.
- I know that things go on behind me. I trust my own intuition and the world around me.
- I am strong, capable, and aware.
- I trust that my inner guides always have my back.

Suggested Stones for the Neck

Aquamarine: For the throat chakra.

Celestite: Known to attract angels. It is a wonderful stone for the throat chakra to be able to call out for what you want.

Angelite: Another blue stone that carries soft, comforting energy and is blue in color. It also attracts angels and helps dispel negative patterns of speech.

Larimar: A wonderful yin stone for mother energy to ease the throat tensions and the neck tensions and help comfort the area with support.

Clear quartz: Helps to clear away any negativity from the body and helps clear and center the recipient. This is a great purifying stone. If you need to clean house of external energies and get down to your own thoughts, this is a great stone to help you do so.

Lapis lazuli: Known for healing the throat chakra and helping with headaches that might stem from tightness in the neck.

Turquoise: Helps with healing of all areas, but helps the neck and throat vibrate to a higher level.

Amazonite: A highly regarded stone to help with the throat chakra as well. This stone honors communication, hope, and trust.

188 | CHAPTER 11

Chrysoprase: A top stone for helping with both physical and energetic neck ailments.

Carnelian: Excellent for the entire back as well as the neck to help ease pains and protect from harm.

Blue lace agate: Helps not only with protection but also with encouragement, higher energies, calming, and elevating.

Labradorite: For transitioning and coming into a higher space where you easily can hold your own energetic space and speak your truth with great ease.

Suggested Essential Oils for Physical Pain

The mint family helps relieve aches and pains.

Peppermint: Reduces inflammation, helps relieve muscle spasms.

Spearmint: Is a less strong version of peppermint with similar if not the same healing properties.

Wintergreen: Is an analgesic like the other mints and helps with spasms and stiffness.

Marjoram: Helps with spasms and increases circulation.

Cypress: Helps relieve muscle spasms.

Blended oils for the purpose of muscle aches is always a good avenue to go for this area of the body as well. When it comes to the mint family and other stimulating oils, it is advised to mix in with a carrier oil and not be applied by itself to the skin. Also a great way to help with neck pain is to take an Epsom salt bath and add any of the above oils or go the other way and add lavender oil to the bath. While it does calm, it also helps physically with muscle spasms.

Suggested Essential Oils for Emotion

This is when you want to focus on the energetics of the neck area. We want to use oils that soothe this area and encourage speaking up, speaking your truth, and being kind. This leans more toward the softer scents:

Rosemary oil: Opens the throat chakra and relieves neck aches. This is especially helpful if you grew up feeling that you were never heard or that you are currently feeling suppressed and having difficulties standing up for yourself.

Lavender: Is a top stress reliever and comforter.

Jasmine: Is an antidepressant scent. Helps to encourage calm, kind, sweet spaces.

Ylang Ylang: Is considered an antidepressant as well as sedative. This oil can help you come into a higher space in your mind as the body calms.

⌘ Flexibility with Life, Love, and Happiness Visualization

You have to know which way is up, which way is in, how to go deep, how to see widely outside of yourself. This visualization will help you to get out of your mundane and realize that just outside of your comfort zone you will see unexpected treasures that await your participation in claiming them.

It is time to go deep within yourself so that you are better able to acknowledge and claim your truth in this life. Who are you? Why are you here? Now is a time in your life to stand up for yourself and claim the divinity that is yours and yours alone. Close your eyes and sit someplace comfortable. Preferably for this meditation, go outside and sit on the ground. Before even thinking deep thoughts, we have to loosen up our necks and our throat chakras so that we can go within and find the answers we may be seeking. Begin by bringing your chin straight down to your chest. Make slow full neck circles; inhale the first half of this circle, moving your left ear to your left shoulder and your head back with your chin facing up to the sky. Exhale as you complete the circle, bringing the right ear to the right shoulder and the chin back down to the chest. Now circle in the opposite direction, to the right this time, inhaling the first half and exhaling the second half.

Each time you get to the front of the chest, change directions but keep the breathing pattern the same. This is a movement from tai chi that helps the neck to unwind itself and match with your breaths. Do this three, six, or nine times in each direction. When you feel your neck is open, bring your head straight ahead and tuck your chin in ever so slightly, opening up the area in the back of the neck at the base of the skull (the jade pillow, as it is referred to). Take deep breaths in through your nose and allow your shoulders to melt down but not slump forward. With each breath in and out feel the tension of the entire body leaving through the soles of your feet, the palms of your hands, out the ear canals, and through your breath. Feel the space between your eyebrows lighten up. Now focus your intention on your neck and your throat. Feel the neck lengthening as the top of your head lifts up like someone is pulling it up by a little string. Get this space open and available to give you the messages it needs you to know.

For this meditation, it's yours. I can't guide you to the questions you seek but I can gently guide the ideas. This is the time that you ask yourself who you are, what you stand for, and if you are willing to stand up for that person and step fully into becoming that person moving forward. This is the time to ask questions and then take at least twice as long in silence to listen for the answers. Too many times when we pray, we ask and we do not wait around long enough to hear the guidance of our souls. This is the time to allow yourself to sit still and wait for answers, images, and thoughts. Don't sift through your thoughts if something random comes in. Just watch and listen and decipher the meanings later.

Be still. Be silent. Be open. Be free.

You deserve to live your best life, and you deserve that best life *right this minute.*

Chapter 12
Putting It All Together to Unlock Your Healing Potential

The ups and downs that come with facing old pains and releasing them is not an easy path to take. Having a deeper awareness of your body, however, can make the process less lonely. As you learn to work with your emotional body rather than against it, the transition will come much more smoothly. Connecting the space between the person you were and the person you are becoming is the purpose of this chapter. This chapter offers insight and tools to help you put it all together.

Years ago, I went to a workshop by an amazing tai chi master. I have been to many workshops that he taught through the years. There are certain people that come in and out of your life and what they come to offer plants a seed that continues to grow long after they return back to where they came from. This particular teacher has taught me so many lessons over the years that I keep tucked away and remember in daily life quite often. There was a day in particular that resonated so deeply with me that I will never forget. The experience taught me a lot about the difference between who I was, and who I was trying to become.

We used to meet down by the Chattahoochee River for our classes and workshops. It was a beautiful space of grass set right beside the water. We spent every weekend for our regular tai chi practice down in that space. But this particular weekend, we had a really special teacher in town. He asked us to each go and find a tree with which we most identified. Go and bond with that tree; figure out why we chose that particular tree. Go spend some time with it. Get connected deeply into the earth energy and the deep roots of your particular tree.

I found this beautiful tree sitting right on the water's edge. It had long, large branches and bright leaves; it seemed so rooted and beautiful. It drew me right to it. I stood near the tree, my feet planted and my body open. I kept looking across the river though to a place with high rocks where some adults were gathered and kids were playing. The side I was on was the quiet side that not that many people knew about. The other side was very public and a whole lot of fun. In fact, the other side of the river where all the people were was exactly where we used to go after school and on weekends when I was in high school. I had a million memories flash up as I looked across the river. Now here I was several years later and in a really hard time in my life. I looked across, wondering how I even got here. How did I get into this place across from that fun place on the other side? How did I wind up with these people and in this crazy tai chi class? When did I stop being the wild party girl I used to be?

I thought deeply about how I could connect the rocks from the old side to this new side that I was now standing on. How I could still have fun like I used to and enjoy life like that party girl, but I now also connect to my deeper, more spiritual side that was developing. The middle of the river was turbulent, just like my mind was. During that time in my life, I was seeking so hard, but I was still so lost and really dealing with a lot of trauma that had come up that I had not yet truly digested and released. It was in that moment of clarity of just how distant the two sides of the river was that I noticed a part of my tree that I had not seen in my initial connection. While the side of the tree that I had seen and ran toward was so beautiful, the other side of the tree, the side that was facing the water, was completely gutted from the inside. It was black, empty, rotting… dying. How did I possibly miss that entire side of this tree? It was exactly a reflection of who I was in that time. I looked the part of the happy, healthy, vibrant girl but inside I was decaying and dying. The decaying and dying part of the tree only showed itself to someone who took the time to come close to the water (or to the real me). I was completely gutted and that tree was the reveal.

When you embark on a spiritual journey, it can feel like you are dropping down the rabbit hole. People that were once huge parts of our lives didn't fit so well anymore. People shift and change and in some cases that means that they leave your life. Going through a spiritual transformation is intensely difficult and unique to each person. I had to work really hard to come back to life fully and reclaim my health, my life, and my healing.

My point of this story is that healing requires you to examine the totality of who you were, who you are, and who you are becoming. Once the initial trauma comes to surface and acknowledged, experienced all over again from a higher perspective, and then finally integrated and transmuted, this is the time when you really have to get to work. One thing we might not realize is that there is comfort in the things we tell ourselves. We get used to those things and, even if it isn't true, if we repeat them enough times, we begin to believe them. We can use this to our advantage in telling ourselves new truths. We can repeat them so many times that we find comfort in the new path as well. You must become vigilant in the fight for the person you are trying to become. It is entirely possible to move into an elevated way of being and continue our lives from that new plane of existence. But we can't just project the ideas, we must become them. We can't just affirm in our healing, we must become healed. *We must live in such a way that there is no other way.*

✿ A Healing Exercise to Lighten the Load

Imagine that you are walking along with a backpack on your back. In the backpack are heavy rocks. Each rock represents something that you experienced that you didn't fully let go of so you packed it up in your backpack and kept on trucking it in forward motion. You don't think much about whatever rock you just threw to the back because it might not have been that big of a deal. It is, however, something you find yourself thinking about often and looking back on and wondering: If it wasn't that big of a deal, why do you keep thinking about it? And so the rock stays in that backpack on your back and you don't even realize it's there. Then you keep doing this time and time again—when you experience a breakup, a loss of any kind, anything that makes you feel bad. You think you dealt with it, and maybe you did for the most part...but is it gone?

With each experience that weighs you down, it literally does weigh you down. It's heavy and you didn't drop it off anywhere. Instead you stuck it in that backpack and kept walking away. Until one day that backpack got so heavy you just couldn't carry it anymore. So you stopped and took a seat and decided to bring that backpack around and have a look inside to see why it has gotten so heavy. You realize that it is full of rocks! How did those even get there? What are they doing there? You've been walking with those rocks for how long now? You are slightly confused how so many rocks piled up, and now you must figure out how to sort through them and then figure out what comes next. You can't keep walking with such a heavy load. Take a seat and pull each stone out one by one.

Next, we must label them. Imagine what your stones would represent, or better yet, collect some actual stones and write the names on them with a marker. Just write down whatever comes to mind as you think of the heavy load that has been dragging you down and holding you back.

Now that we have begun the process of sorting through and separating feelings and experiences, this does not end there. You have to go through the memory banks in your mind of each and every stone and actually re-experience it, but as if you are watching it through a movie screen. Watch closely, let yourself feel the emotions, but also let yourself become the narrator instead of the lead character. You know that's you…but somehow, it's not you anymore. You allow yourself to see this situation through a clearer picture and through the eyes that do not stay in that space and are not overly attached to the outcome but more insightful to what it has done to you since. How do you help yourself now? Get a game plan of healing each and every one of these stones and what they meant to you. This does not have to all be addressed in one sitting. This can be done one stone at a time, one stone a day, or several at a time, depending on importance once you sort them out.

If you are writing things down and labeling the rocks, be sure to follow up after addressing each stone with a new word of how you feel about the situation before releasing the rock completely. Compare the two words, the initial feeling and label to the newer word, once you have worked your way through and out of whatever it was to begin with. We've all been in relationships where at the time we were absolutely devastated and could not see the bigger picture. Everyone in their life should have at least one soul-crushing, devastating heartbreak so you can be a much better partner later for a much better person. It's a necessary heartbreak for soul growth. At the time though, it's easy to get super lost in it and let the pain and loss eat you up and take away your self-worth. Anytime someone chooses to leave you, you are left wondering what is wrong with you. Somehow we don't question anything larger than that. But now that you've had some time under your belt, looking back might make you smirk and giggle at the absurdity that was that relationship. So the label might have started with devastated or left behind or dumped or crushed, while the new label now that you have healed through and seen it for what it was might be labeled: learning lesson, never again, silly, growth, peaceful.

These rocks tell your story—let your story be told to you again in such a way that you are no longer attached to the endings of any of them. If you are writing it all down, once you have completed the exercises, set that piece of paper on fire and let it turn to ash. Leave all of those rocks back there and walk forward with an empty backpack on your back. You'll still throw things into that backpack as you move along, but it won't be any of the same things from back then.

This exercise should be done many times along the journey of your life for proper introspection and healing. Too many times we catch ourselves weighed down with a super heavy backpack, but now you can be more conscious of this action and start cleaning house much earlier than you have done before.

A Lesson in Forgiveness

Forgiveness is something that is vital in your healing process. It is something that is extremely difficult to do but must be applied to the emotional traumas that may still be sitting within your being. This way you can move on with your life in a much more positive and loving way. Our emotional bodies will heal in miraculous ways when we learn to forgive not necessarily the person or situation, but the role that we play and the attachment to its effects.

I have a dear friend who graduated from seminary with a master of divinity degree. She is a combination of ordained minister, endorsed chaplain, Reiki master, meditation instructor, student of world religions, and so much more. She specializes in addiction medicine and has been the spiritual counselor for some world-renowned drug and alcohol treatment centers. She teaches a course on forgiveness. Forgiveness is a key that unlocks a great amount of pain and long-standing tension in your whole body and mind. It is very powerful, and I've asked her to share the basics of it with us. We could all use a lesson in forgiveness if we are sincerely committed to healing ourselves and our lives. The way she described to me with regard to forgiveness as a part of our daily lives was this: "For me, forgiveness is the practice of remembering a painful event, accepting that it happened as it did, and letting go of my attachment to it and the pain it caused. It is not forgetting, condoning, tolerating, enabling, or self-sacrificing. It is accepting and letting go. It is an act of self-love." (Please see appendix B for a full exercise from Ashli on forgiveness.)

Next Steps to the Process: Being Present with Your Emotions

You will need to learn how to acclimate to your newly lightened emotional body. Too many times we feel so naked without our pain that we quickly summon it back to us. It makes us feel vulnerable and raw to remove the pain and learn to trust in our own happiness. That is the scariest part of it all. We wait for the other shoe to drop. Therefore, we must get to work quickly to close up the new hole where the roots of the carrots once were (I call the deeply rooted pains "carrots" because they grow down deep just like the carrots in your garden). Remember that these pains and deep roots took many years to create and dig deep into our energy bodies. We first feel immediate relief and bliss having them removed, and then the reality sets in that we don't know what to do with that new space. It can feel raw and exposed. We have created a life where that pain is such a part of us that to be without it is really uncomfortable.

First we must treat the physical part of this new process. We must acknowledge that rawness and feel it and go deeply into it—not away from it. You can't just cover it up real quick and run. Dive down into it and feel all that is so raw and exposed. Let your body feel it. Let your body feel what is now missing, let it feel what was removed, let it feel the sheer nakedness of feeling so completely opened up.

With any physical injury, the fibroblasts lay themselves over the injured area and create scar tissue. They lie every which way over the trauma in hopes to heal it quickly. When it comes to emotional traumas, we quickly face the parts we can and tuck the rest away for another day. But the body's energy healers—much like the fibroblasts—will try their best to cover it up quickly to help you move on. Then underneath, if left untreated, the shadows below grow and root down while you are busy doing other things. As you go through this book and apply the practice to yourself for healing, you cannot afford to let anything dig deeper without you noticing. You must be willing to race against this process and get to it first so there is no planting of shadow roots within. Go deep and jump all the way down the rabbit hole. Come back up renewed.

⌘ Visualization for Being Present

Imagine a garden with carrots all in a row. Lie down next to the carrots so that they are next to each chakra in your body. As you go through your whole energy system, gently reach down to the root and pull the full carrot up and out of your garden. Pair these carrots with your thoughts on what you are willing to let go of and then take each thought out of your garden, root by root. Then lay the carrots down as an offering for the bunnies to eat. (Bunnies as animal messages represent fear. Give them your fear. You are free.)

Visit the pains and where they came from. Let yourself time travel and feel it all over again, but this time, lead yourself back up and out. We don't do that during trauma. We don't know how. The waves that will come over you again and again today and through the night will be hard to feel, but you must and it is important to be clear of mind in this space. You have to feel it. Let yourself be sad and mad and shame-filled and resentful and whatever other emotions come up for you. Be honest about them, and be sad with them. Grieve with them all. Give yourself permission to just go down into the deep for as long as you possibly need to be down there, then pull up from the root each carrot that represents each painful, old space. This part won't last forever, but it is one of the most important steps you can do to truly heal and be free to move forward without the burdens.

Once we pull those carrots out, let's fill each open space with a splendid healing color of our choice. Feel what color resonates with that area and pour it in like a hot liquid. Watch it crystallize. Green represents healing, blue represents trust and calm, yellow can mean trust and softness, and orange brings in creative joys. Purple is a wonderful color to bring in healing light of a regal nature. White and gold are the ultimate healing colors of purity and grace. See in your mind what colors are being requested by the energy of the new open space and pour it in.

Envision any of the colors that you choose turning into an opaque, shiny color that melts right into each place perfectly, closing the area with incredibly clean healing properties. Stay in this space for as long as you need to. When you are ready, slowly wiggle your fingers and toes. Move your body slowly and become aware of the air on your skin. Do a full body scan and make sure that the fillings are perfectly in line with the rest of your energy body. Come out of this visualization feeling healed and new.

Where Does the Good Stuff Go?

Practically everything that is discussed in healing always revolves around clearing the body of negative emotions: trauma, shame, guilt, fear, anger, sadness. But where does the good stuff go? Life is not all a series of emotional traumas that get stored in the mind and affect the brain and body.

Healing exists. Miracles exist too. We understand that in the mind there are grooves that represent our thought patterns. The way that we think and perceive things affects those grooves, and we understand that through positive thinking we can change those mind grooves into something that is healthier and better for us. We hear about visualization and the way that meditations and affirmations along with visualization can help to heal. Mostly attributed to Ivan Pavlov's research, we have learned that responses that the body has forgotten can be brought back by repetition. Although maybe not as strong, it can be recovered psychologically. The mind and the muscles store emotion—not only emotions of trauma, but also emotions of joy, love, and bliss. Those higher emotions must too be stored in the same way as the traumas.

But how does the mind process the good emotions and thoughts and the chemicals? And how do the muscles react? There's not a lot of research on this because nobody seems to focus on the good stuff. All that good stuff gets absorbed into muscle memory, but does it store itself in the mind and the muscles in the same way that the trauma emotions do? And if it does process the same way and it is sitting in the same spaces, then how do we utilize this knowledge for our greatest health?

Emotional release, trauma, and shame and all the other darker emotions have to have their light counterparts. The muscle memory also stores the good things. Even if we return to an exercise that we hadn't done in so long, our muscles rejoice! They remember!

But it isn't just exercise that they pull back up and remember, it is also the emotions that came along with those happier and more active times in our lives.

How many of us miss terribly the days when we were cheerleaders or soccer players or runners or anything from the school days that involved athletics? My friend invented a program for cheerleaders and cheer enthusiasts called PoundPoms™. It uses weighted pom poms to bring back the old cheerleading days but into the gyms and senior centers and adult exercise places of any kind. What if we always wanted to be a cheerleader but never could? Now there is a workout specifically for the fun that came along with cheerleading with a light weight added, no uniform needed, and it's just to make our bodies have fun while doing something healthy. Her mother teaches her fitness class with the PoundPoms™ at her local senior center. They love it! They laugh and play and dance around while getting a great workout in.

But is it more than that? Is it more than just the love of cheerleading and feeling young again? Is it that your muscles also rejoice as they go back in time and do motions from some of the best times in their life? It came so easy back then, and it was so much fun! And what chemicals are releasing from the brain as you do return to these mighty movements? We experience actual joy in movement as we do the motions. Mental pictures in your mind replaying good or hard memories of the good old days. Are you dancing and cheering while creating emotional bliss? Think about how this affects the muscle/mind connection. This has to be such a treat for the body to get to go back in time to a place where you were at your peak in youth in performance and social life! What joy it brings to me when I get to go play this way and bring my muscles and my mind back to such an incredible time of my life. She figured out how to make exercise fun again for us! We sweat, we cry, we laugh, we embrace as our body moves and rekindles the romance with your own muscles and connection to the mind.

Find your favorite inspirational song or a song that reminds you of the greatest time in your life. Whatever your theme song was during a high time or even a low time if you want to use it to heal. Turn it up high and dance. Dance in a way that softens your body and lets those old energetic bubbles pop out from each joint of your body as you move about. Let the energy collect and explode off each fingertip and out from the soles of your feet. Get into the lyrics. Sync up with the rhythm. Lighten any lines on your face as you discover movement as a way to release pain.

Using the Good Stuff for Your Own Healing

We've explored throughout this book some of the ways in which the muscles contain memory. They contain memory for any simple physical movement, and they contain memory of emotions that the mind has stored within them. The upside of all this is that the muscles remember what they are like when they are healthy. Even if in your mind it might not be as memorable, the memory of good health, of joy, of happiness—all that is stored within the muscles, and this resource can be tapped into and utilized for your own healing. Spontaneous healing does happen. Your body remembers being healthy. Trust your body more and pull from within its stored memories to heal you. It's not all about releasing. It's about pulling from within and being reminded of the good stuff, and then changing patterns and habits within yourself to get back to that better space of greater positivity and wellness in real time.

You can heal yourself. Your muscles and your mind are the key masters. Whether the healing comes through faith, through answered prayer, or from an incredible surgery or any other treatment strategy, your body must be part of the conversation in order for you to heal completely and move forward. Remember *the body heals itself*. However, it does not heal without your full participation. It's a formula and only you will know what yours will be. You have to listen to your muscles, your mind, your gut, and your heart. Think of it as a jury. If one of those things votes the other way, there is chaos. You have to do the work to create and establish peace within your whole being. Once they are all playing on the same side, you just may get your miracles.

❀ FINAL MEDITATION

This meditation is intended to bring you back to yourself, coming into the simplicity of being fully present to yourself and your life. Close your eyes and take a deep breath in and out. Clear your mind; calm your body through your breath and through intention to do so. Place one hand over your heart and feel its sacred rhythm through each beat. That is purpose. Tune into your purpose in this life. Place the other hand on your solar plexus. That's instinct. Trust the purpose that your heart has for this life. Go deeper and feel the pulse of each cell in your body. Tune into the sacred intelligence that your cells carry through you. Allow these to show you your soul's desire. Listen intently to what your purpose, instincts, and body's intelligence have to say to you. Sit still, be calm, and listen to the call from deep within. Stay in this space for as long as it takes to listen to your inner wisdom. Take it to heart.

Once you come out of this space (slowly and with intention) begin to let the messages your body has given to you resonate and take shape. Tune into your soul's purpose and begin to make small yet meaningful changes toward creating your very best and most purposeful life. It's yours for the making. Trust that you have everything in you to make it come alive.

Affirmations

For this affirmation exercise, don't choose just one. Say them all.

- In this moment, every cell in my body corrects itself. Every strand of DNA is recomposed, straightened, and healed.
- Any parts of me that have been out of balance restore themselves *now*.
- I am healed at the deepest cellular level.
- I agree to move forward while trusting my body, my heart, and my mind.
- I am now able to live the life I have always imagined I could.
- I ask that this be so … And So It Is.

Miracles happen every day. You are allowed to have yours, too.

Additional Tools to Try
Cleanse, Release, Ground, and Empower

Now that you know more about the emotions that are stored within your muscle body, it's time to gain some additional tools you can use to help you in your own healing. In this section, you'll discover tools and techniques to cleanse, release, ground, and empower.

To Cleanse

Taking time out to cleanse yourself not just physically but emotionally is extremely important. There are simple things that you can do to help you align your body-mind in a soft way that frees itself of the heaviness of stagnant chi.

A great way to cleanse your energy is to take a bath. Water cleanses our physical bodies as well as our emotional and energy bodies. You can add herbs, oils, salts, and other ingredients to your recipes to really help draw those toxins out of the body to leave you feeling purified and refreshed. Here are some recipes to try:

Bath to Nourish

1–2 cups Epsom salt

1–2 cups sea salt

5–10 drops lavender and/or rosemary fresh

Milk Bath

Rose petals help you remember things. Placing rose petals under the pillow at night will help you remember your dreams. Rose is also a wonderful bath tool that can be mixed in with the water for a special, loving, nourishing, soul-soothing, body-soothing experience when added to any bath. You can use dry rose petals and crumple them into small bits easier to get down the drain, or feel free to use fresh full rose petals intact.

A nice addition to the rose petals is to add some warm milk (goats milk is best but any milk of your choice is fine). Milk helps to break up any oils on the skin. Let a candle burn nearby for full effect as you relax in the bath.

Goddess Bath

Dried oats

Goat's milk, powdered buttermilk, or powdered cow milk

Dried flowers like lavender, rose, calendula, and/or chamomile

Essential oils of chamomile, orange, rose petal, tea rose, and/or lavender

Place these in a sachet and drop into the tub, or add water to make a paste and use as a facial or body scrub.

To Release

The key to a detox bath is what comes after the actual bath. Fill the tub with at least one cup of salt. I prefer one to two cups of sea salt and one to two cups of Epsom salt. Fill the tub as hot as you are comfortable in so that you begin to create a sweat. Stay in the tub as long as you can, ideally ten to fifteen minutes.

Now for the real part. Wrap yourself in a towel and stay in that towel. Get under the covers, even pull the comforter all the way up to your chin and tuck your arms underneath as well. Now you will sweat it out. Stay in that towel under the sheets for as long as you can possibly handle it. Usually ten to fifteen minutes, but don't time it. You are the timer. There will come a moment where you will kick off those covers and you will not be able to stand one more minute of this sweating hotness! That is when you are finished with your detox. Keep a lot of water by you and drink at least one full glass, preferably one while in the tub and one after the sweat.

Once you are done with your detox, feel free to jump in the shower to rinse off. I recommend only doing this at night because you will feel quite weak after this experience. I personally do this detox after receiving any bodywork—massage, chiropractic, acupuncture, Reiki—anything where your body will need to adjust itself to release things that have been moved around and brought up.

Basic Detox Bath

2 cups Epsom salt

1–2 cups sea salt

1 pinch to a full cup of baking soda (aluminum-free)

1 cup bentonite clay (optional)

5–10 drops lavender or another essential oil of your choice (be sure it's an oil that is non-toxic and safe for the skin)

Sacred Clay Detox Bath

Green Aztec Clay is a wonder clay, especially when you add apple cider vinegar to it to create the perfect paste to put on your face, neck, hands, and any other part of your body that you need to help pull out the toxins. Put it on until it dries and then shower first and then choose from one of the above baths to follow up with. Or make your own bath scrub to remove the clay in the shower.

Sugar Scrub

Skin scrubs can be very cleansing as they help slough away that dull outer layer. Use these scrubs to help you feel relaxed and revitalized. Use fine or coarse granulated sugar (depending on personal preference. I personally like fine salt or sugar for a body scrub) and mix with a carrier oil like jojoba, coconut, grapeseed oil, avocado oil (more expensive but awesome), or olive oil. Add five to fifteen drops of essential oil.

For Grounding: Sandalwood, rosewood, cedarwood, patchouli, frankincense, myrrh are great choices to add to the sugar scrub.

For Relaxing: Lavender, ylang ylang, jasmine, rose, neroli are all great options for the relaxing finish. Opening to love, feeling love, relaxing, and healing are these scents.

For Revitalizing: Peppermint, spearmint, wintergreen, rosemary, eucalyptus (in very small amount because it's not advised to be on skin unless with serious carrier oils as recommended).

Salt Scrub

It is the exact same as the sugar scrub but instead of fine granulated sugar, use fine or coarse salt, depending on preference, or sea salt.

To Ground—Earthing

If what you need is to get grounded and centered and back into your body fully, look no further than your own backyard. Get those shoes off and get outside onto the earth! Walk around in the dirt, the mud, the grass, just nothing cement. Become aware of your steps; become aware of what you are stepping on. Become aware of the trees around you and maybe go touch one, sit with one, or dare I say it…hug one. Get grounded, let Mother Earth heal your heart, and your body. Let the sacred waves and pulse of the earth enter through your feet and up into your whole being. Breathe deeply and fully and clear away the clutter of your mental thoughts. Do not bring your phone out with you. No electrical devices of any kind come along on this ride. Get serious, go within, and don't come back in until you've settled whatever is scattered within.

Mixing Heaven and Earth

This breathing practice is especially helpful when you are doing your earthing outside, but anywhere will do for this experience. Spread the feet hip width apart and soften the knees and hips. Let the arms hang down long and exhale all of your breath. Then as you turn your palms up and lift your arms up and over your head, take a slow, deep inhale. Take in through your hands energy from the heavens. Then as you exhale, bring the arms down with your fingertips facing each other but not touching. Bring the energy down through the front of the body and down over the top of the head, over the chest, stomach, down through the legs, and through the feet into the earth as you exhale. Imagine your legs are like a tree and then breathe deeply into the roots beyond the earth's surface. That is how far the exhale and the energy should be going. Do this at least three times. Inhale, take in the energy from the heavens. Exhale, bring the energy into your upper dantian (energy center at the third eye), middle dantian (energy at the solar plexus), and the lower dantian (below the navel to the sacral chakra). In Tai Chi Chuan, this is where the body is believed to hold its strongest energy.

To Empower

The sacred art of breathing. Want to change your life? Change your breath. Where there is breath, there is life and there is hope and anything is possible. In my yoga training, my teacher would say that you can cause or cure disease through the breath. When we are stressed out, depressed, anxious, or shame-filled, our breathing changes and can manifest illness. When we are cleaned out, rejuvenated, balanced, healthy, and happy, our breath is from a deeper place in our lower bellies and diaphragm. It can help to rectify our current state of health. Here are some breathing practices for healing:

Pranayama

Just when you thought you knew how to breathe, you enter either a tai chi/chi gong or yoga class and find out you have had it wrong ever since you broke the correct cycle of breathing that only babies seem to know. I don't know if it happens during adolescence when we are told to suck in or when it exactly switches to the opposite way of breathing correctly for life and longevity, but I've never encountered anyone who did not need re-teaching of this very natural way of being. When we inhale, our bellies should expand out like a balloon. When we exhale, we bring the navel back toward the spine. Here are some very easy techniques to help you develop single-pointed focus, enhance blood circulation and quality of the blood, as well as make you healthier and happier.

Relaxation Breathing

This is a breathing technique that absolutely every person should know. It's the easiest of any pranayama techniques. Relaxation breath is all about breathing from your belly and not from your chest. Inhale and let your belly expand like a balloon. Exhale and let the air out, bringing the navel back toward the spine. When you inhale, pay attention to your shoulders, they should not rise up with your breath. This is a tension breathing pattern, and we want to rid you of this as soon as possible.

Becoming aware of this easy breathing will be the first step to reverse the tension breaths that everyone somehow learns along the way. The tension breath becomes a part of you when sucking in your gut becomes a part of your awareness. This all of a sudden changes up the breathing. If you approach anyone who has never had directive breathing lessons and you ask them to take a deep breath, their shoulders rise up, you can hear them breathe in so deep that you would think they were about to jump off a diving board into a pool. Then on the exhale it too is loud and doesn't really release. It's all up in the chest and shoulders, and this is painful and unhealthy.

Let your stomach come out with a breath in. It only makes sense that the stomach expands when oxygen enters—exactly like a balloon. But when people get self-conscious about their stomachs, they suck them in and then the breath only goes upward and not outward. Then they are only breathing from a very small space within their lung capacity, making it harder to fully oxygenate your blood and have a healthy mind and body. Stressful short breaths can easily lead to high blood pressure and other out-of-balance stresses within the body. Relax into it; let it open. Keep the shoulders down, just move with your belly and make the exhale count. Don't focus on a big breath in; focus on a bigger breath out.

Full Yogic Breath

The diaphragm is responsible for 80 percent of your full lung capacity. The next 10 percent is from your sternum (center of the chest) and the remaining 10 percent is from the clavicle (collarbones). If you bring your arms down by your sides and lift the arms straight up with an inhale, without even having to think about it you expand through the diaphragm, the sternum, and the clavicle to give you a full breath, utilizing 100 percent of the lungs' capacity. When you exhale, bring the arms straight back down and it will unload in the same way. I love to do this in bed several times upon waking or before going to sleep. You can do this sitting, standing, or lying down. Let the arms lead the way and let the movement be in sync to the speed of the breath. This is so simple to do and so effective. If you are feeling stressed out, anxious, or depressed, this is the perfect thing to excuse yourself and go to the bathroom and do. Just stand upright against a wall and bring the arms all the way up with the inhale. Bring them straight back down with the exhale. Do this at least five rounds.

Ujjayi Breathing

This sort of breathing sounds a lot like Darth Vader if you do it correctly. It is different than other breathing techniques in that it is done paired with actual motion, specifically yoga asanas. There is a slight constriction in the back of your throat during the exhales. As you go forward, the constricting and deep sound can be practiced through both the inhale and the exhale. It is a deep *AHHHH* sound but with the lips tightly shut. A place deep down to bring the breath up and out. It cleanses the body and rids it of toxins. This breath enhances body heat and is excellent to do while engaging in energy work as well to keep your body clean and available for the highest vibrational energy possible to come through. Ujjayi breathing increases energy, and it brings the awareness to a center point throughout the body and mind. Many refer to this breath as ocean breathing.

Alternate Nostril Breathing

This breathing is good for focusing on the third eye and balancing the brain. There are different hand positions for this practice, but I am keeping it to the third eye for this. I am also not holding any breaths for this, but in my yoga practice we inhale for four, hold the breath for sixteen, and exhale for a count of eight. For this practice, I will teach it for beginners and for simple purposes of just inhaling and exhaling.

Sit comfortably with your spine straight. Keep your chin in and slightly down. Take your right hand and cross your index and middle finger and place those fingers at the third eye. Inhale through the left nostril and then close both nostrils for a moment. Exhale through the right nostril. Then inhale through that right nostril and close both nostrils for a moment. Exhale through the left nostril. Inhale left and then hold. Exhale right and inhale right and then hold. Exhale left. We begin and finish on the left side. One full round looks like this:

- Exhale both nostrils to begin
- Inhale left
- Close the nostrils
- Exhale right
- Inhale right

- Close the nostrils
- Exhale left
- That completes one full round.

Aim for four to six full rounds. Once you have taken your last exhale through the left side, lower your hands down and breath deeply and easily through both nostrils, keeping your eyes closed so you can allow your body to feel how open and balanced the breath is now. Come out of this slowly and enjoy those moments of being fully focused on something. That is your gateway to meditation.

Nostril Breathing

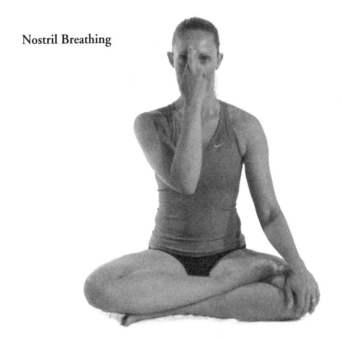

Angel Breathing

Begin sitting in a cross-legged, comfortable position that allows your spine to be straight, your hips to be open, and your neck to be comfortable. Clasp your hands together under your chin with your elbows touching or as close as they can be. Exhale all of your breath. Inhale as you lift the elbows up and out like wings as your chin opens up to the ceiling, keeping your hands still clasped underneath. As the elbows or wings open fully, so do the lungs in that one giant inhale. As you exhale, bring the elbows back together and slowly back down along with your chin to the starting position. Repeat this several times. Feel your lungs as your wings expand, feeling clearly open and free with each inhale. Bring the head up and back, keep your eyes closed. As you return the elbows and the chin down, always keeping the hands just under the chin, feel the energy come back to center with a warming, calming, centering experience. Grounding with each exhale back into center and in close like a child. Freeing, soaring, opening, expanding, and loving with each inhale. Embrace the heavens and the earth in your inhale. Embrace the earth and your inner child with each exhale. Be free with this breath, let it take your mind where it wants. Be open and embrace all.

Angel Breathing—Part 1

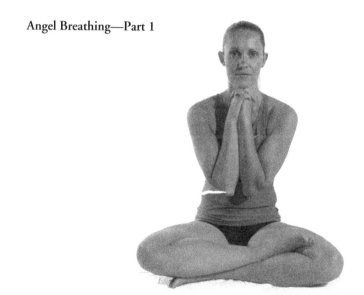

Angel Breathing—Part 2

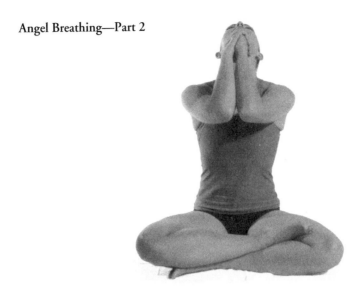

Angel Breathing—Part 3

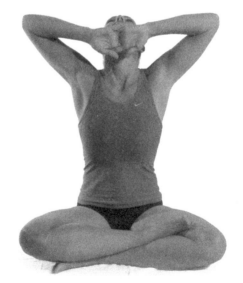

Communing with Spirit

Sit up comfortably with the spine straight, the chin slightly tucked in but not down. The palms face up and rest on your knees or in your lap. Close your eyes and relax your face. Imagine that God, Great Spirit, or whatever you want to refer to it as is now either over you or in front of you. You will exchange breaths with spirit. Your exhale is God's inhale. When God exhales, it's your inhale. Focus only on the energy between you and Spirit. Every breath you exchange goes in through you, out through them, in through them, and out through you. Stay in this space for as long as you are able to feel it and see it in your mind's eye. You will notice quickly that everything else around you falls away and a single-pointed focus directly with Great Spirit is happening. Be sure when you end this exchange to give thanks.

To Purify the Blood

This is a genetic predisposition, so it either comes totally naturally for you or it never will. Take the tongue and fold it in on both sides to make a tub or a taco with it. Inhale through your tongue and exhale through your nose. Repeat this at least ten rounds to help purify the blood.

Stones

As we covered various crystals and stones throughout this book, I want to offer specific stones for additional emotions. Stones can be worn as jewelry on the body or placed on your body loosely while you are lying down. They can be placed underneath the bed, in your pockets, or around your home. Anywhere you are, stones are always helpful if you know which ones to get for your specific purpose.

Best Stone to Help with Loss

The Apache tear is absolutely the best stone to have for loss. Especially if you lost someone because they died. This stone is a powerful healing stone and assists with extreme sadness and loss. They are strong grounding stones and provide protection. Use this as an aid to clear negative emotions that may be holding you back.

The legend behind the Apache tear: seventy-five brave Apache warriors were attacked by soldiers of the US army. Of the seventy-five men, fifty were killed at the hands of the army. The remaining warriors decided to jump off the cliff to their deaths rather than be killed by the soldiers. The women and children that were left behind by the warriors began to weep. Their tears hit the ground and turned to stone—the Apache tear stone. The legend says that those who carry this stone don't have to cry anymore, because the women and children cried enough for all who mourn. It is believed that these stones have great spiritual and healing power because of this. The Apache tear stone is a form of obsidian.

Fairy Crosses are also incredible stones for healing through loss and have a similar story behind them. The legend is at the time that Christ was crucified, the fairies cried and their tears turned to stones. Those stones are in the shape of a cross but never a perfect cross because of the imperfections of human nature.

Best Stone to Help with Renewal

The green stones are considered master stones for renewal and connection to the higher spaces of consciousness. Stones like green tourmaline and green calcite both connect to the heart center. Moldavite is an excellent stone. It is a very powerful stone and not of this earth. You must be ready to wear something so powerful. It connects you to the cosmos and helps to strengthen and restore your own sacred energy. Use your intention and ask for affirmation if moldavite is the right stone for you.

Crystals for Protection, Clearing, and Healing

Amethyst: A great stone for love and to relieve pain.

Apophyllite: This stone will keep your energy separate from the clients. It is a beautiful protector stone.

Aventurine: A stone for love that also helps with the back, the spine, and the heart channels and the heart center.

Bloodstones: Always smart to have on hand as well, since they have to do with immunity. This helps increase the immune system. People even put bloodstone in their water to help increase the immunity of the water so you can ingest it and have that energy inside the body. Obviously, do not eat any stones themselves.

Citrine: Encourages joy and abundance. This stone oftentimes is used to attract money and dispel fears of not having enough.

Clear quartz: Always a great cleanser stone.

Desert Rose: It is made of selenite, and it is considered a wishing stone. If you can get your hands on a desert rose you make one wish with it, but afterward you must return it to the earth. Burying it or throwing it into water (although water makes the stone dissolve) as your trade for your wish and intention to manifest.

Fluorite: Comes in a lot of color combos. Generally, it has stripes of green and purple and clear colors. Fluorite is a good soothing stone. Soothing illnesses and calming the body. Known to speed healing. Fluorite is a great protection stone from other people's energies and emotions. Can help with better sleep and to protect from bad dreams.

Girasol opal: Another powerful stone to have on hand. In fact, two for this is better than one. One for each hand. These stones help you tell the truth. I like to put one of these in each of the client's hands if they are blocked. They need to release, they want to release, but honestly they have blocked so much out of their deeper consciousness that a little help is needed. The girasol opal helps to bring old truths, real truths, and hidden truths to the surface. My acupuncturist uses this stone a lot in her practice working with people who have serious illness to help them uncover their own pains and shames.

Green tourmaline: A stone for love and protection of the lungs and heart as well as healing energy for the wearer or recipient.

Hematite: A grounding, earthy stone. Although I've never seen it in the books, my teacher said not to wear hematite around the neck as it blocks the heart energy and keeps you separated from loving energies. He preferred to put hematite on wrists and ankles when on your person, or put it at the foot of any bed or table to help increase the earth energy. I see many hematite necklaces as jewelry. I'm sure it's fine, but personally, I keep to his advice and only wear it as bracelets or anklets. I have found in times where my energy was way too flighty, putting on all four has brought me back down in a healthy way.

Jade: A stone of earth energy, grounding, and support to the wearer.

Kyanite: Used to balance the chakras, but it needs to be cleaned thoroughly if someone other than yourself is using it.

Moonstone: The stone of the woman. Also a stone that will need to be cleaned well and often if you are sharing it.

Obsidian: In my opinion, obsidians of any kind in energy/healing work is not the top choice. Obsidians tend to magnify whatever you are feeling. Therefore, if the feelings are not strong and supple, the energy basically doubles with obsidian stones. It's a great stone to have, but not as a top choice in bodywork. I do have a very rare obsidian called a green sheen obsidian. It is heavy and large and it pulls out the negative energy from the body. I never let any other person touch that stone. Since it is to pull out the negative, place it on your chest with a rose quartz above it on the chest and a clear quartz at the top of the head. It must be laid out in this pattern. I use it when I've had a hard day or feel overwhelmed or anxious and let the heavy stone sit on my chest. When I was going through a really hard time I would use it and somehow always fall into a deep meditation or sleep. It really brought about some very deep, heavy emotions but knowing that I could direct the energy out of my heart space and into this stone was and continues to be extremely helpful. When it comes to laying stones… nothing is set in stone except for the actual stones themselves. There are no hard and fast rules. The rules I've been given don't match someone else's rules that they have been given. You first learn the basics and read the books and then you start learning from the stones themselves and follow the guidance you get directly from communication and intuition.

Rhodochrosite: This stone consists of shades of pink. It has more to do with intense self-love. Like rhodonite, it too is a heart space, loving stone but the focus is from within and around your own being. It has more to do with child energy of your own and helps you to release old patterns and embrace new loving patterns.

Rhodonite: A pink and black colored stone that is a powerful heart center stone. Rhodonite, according to my stone teacher, varies from the rhodochrosite in that if you see the black in it, it is a rhodonite, which is for universal loving, heart-centered energy. It is also a great emotional balancer and stress-relieving stone.

Rose quartz: Keeps unconditional love as its primary.

Snowflake Obsidian: Is an excellent tool for grounding your energy or anyone else's.

Smokey quartz: My top choice for clearing away energies.

Combination of stones: Clear quartz, rose quartz, fluorite, bloodstone, and amethyst. Those five are a wonderful basic cleaning group of stones. I like to put that concoction into water as well, especially for my pets. If you choose to use this group of stones and put them in water to drink, be sure the stones are large enough that you don't choke on them and do not consume them. The stones infuse the water. Also, stones should only be placed in either glass or wood but not metal of any kind and especially no plastic.

To Clean Your Stones

Crystals absorb energy, therefore it is important to keep your stones clean. Here are some ways to wash your stones and clear them of people's energies:

Placing the stones out under the full moon for the night is one of the best ways to clean them. Also, washing them with water and light soap is good. I like to do this before I lay them out under the moon for the night. Putting the stones in sea salt if they are small enough to be covered well is always easy and great. Smudge your stones. Smudge everything—you can never have too much sage love in your life. You can also clean the stones through your own intentions. Place your hands on the stones and give prayer, affirmations, and intentions to clean the stones of any and all energies.

Additional Modalities to Try
Various Offerings on Avenues to Healing

Western medicine is allopathic and tends to focus more on the symptoms. Eastern medicine focuses more on the whole person and the root cause. Eastern medicine encompasses traditional Chinese/Japanese medicine (acupuncture and herbs), as well as Ayurvedic medicine (medicine practiced in India). This section will introduce Eastern philosophies of healing. I highly encourage you to search outside your comfort zone if your body is in need of correction. No one person can be an expert in every field. Therefore, I have reached out to people who specialize in these different areas for the purpose of this book.

The purpose of this section is to give you a wider view of opportunities for healing. There are so many ways to heal out there and so many options if you know what to look for and what resonates with you or whoever you are trying to help. I think it is vital when you are trying to heal to know that there are other opportunities out there that might be a better fit if you are willing to give them a try. Remember, your ability to heal is so much greater than you may have ever been taught to believe. In order to do this, you must widen the lens. This means look outside of the standard health-care practices and take a dip into how the other half lives.

This is a collection of interviews that I introduced throughout the book for additional avenues and information.

Ayurvedic Medicine

Aryuveda is a Sanskrit word meaning "the complete knowledge for long life." It's about how you *digest* every aspect of your life. Because Ayurveda is so incredibly intense even in its explanation, I went in search of a top practitioner who had the skills and the knowledge to give a proper introduction of this sacred healing tradition. I went to people I knew from Kripalu, the mecca of yoga, meditation, and Ayurvedic body treatments located in the Berkshires, and found Laura Spucches. I asked her to explain Ayurveda in a way we could all easily understand. Below is her offering:

How Ayurveda Is in Relation to "Issues in the Tissues" by Laura Spucches

When it comes to solving issues in the tissues, Ayurveda has more than 5,000 years of experience under its belt. Rather than a one-size-fits-all approach to healing, Ayurveda's multidimensional view abides natural law by viewing each individual's "issues" through an elemental lens. When the fundamental elements (ether, air, fire, water, earth) go out of balance, this can lead to disease. Highly trained practitioners who understand these fundamentals of the science of life go through each individual's life with a fine-toothed comb in order to understand not only the lifestyle and diet of the individual but the external factors and the internal spirit, in order to understand where the imbalance first occurred. They then take the root causative factors, gently shift or remove them, and add in the other components to suit your individual needs.

When we first understand the individual's elemental makeup—vata being ether and air, pitta being fire and water, kapha being water and earth—and the imbalances that have occurred over the duration of the individual's life, Ayurveda employs appropriate Chikitsas or treatments to help the individual to attain balance within the mind, body, and spirit. The treatments can range from a simple shift in lifestyle or diet to a complete thirty, sixty, ninety+ days turnaround through panchakarma (the five actions of purification and retreat).

Over time, the body absorbs its environment from the foods that we choose to the music that we listen to through the people that we choose to associate with. It's the good old saying "we are what we eat" or even "you tell me what you've been eating (including all sensory input) and I'll tell you who you are!" As humans, we basically "eat" life! Our sensory experience of this natural world forms our experience and eventually our tissues.

All of our choices and experiences have impacts on our overall health and well-being, making everything that we do, touch, taste, smell, hear, choose not to do, have done to us either our medicine or our poison.

A completely healthy and balanced person should be able to process anything that comes into the body and mind with ease. This assumes that the individual's agni (Ayurvedic term for fire—the digesting principle) and baseline constitution have remained in balance throughout the seasons, throughout the shifts of life from childhood to adulthood (hormonal years) and right through to the wisdom years (non-hormonal years) of life. But for the overwhelming majority of people issues get stuck.

According to Ayurveda, what this really means is that there is a certain level of ama (or undigested stuff) occurring within the existence of the individual. Therefore, how well we digest our food, our experiences, and our environment matters! Every facet of everything that occurs within, throughout, and around our general being has to be digested and digested properly in order for the proper formation of healthy physiological tissues. How often have you gone to a relative's house and had a disagreement that you just couldn't get over for days, weeks, or months? And how often have those issues "stuck," not only in your mind but maybe affected your sleep, which then began the roller-coaster ride into health-related issues?

Our ability to properly digest and assimilate our lives' "food" will ultimately determine our mind, body, and emotional outcomes. Therefore, Ayurveda, with its more than 5,000 years of life knowledge, has been focused on how well we digest and assimilate our food. If our digestion within our GI tract is balanced and in tip-top shape… not too strong and not too weak… this allows the body to properly process and assimilate all of nature's elemental knowledge, helping support the entire system and keep it balanced throughout the cycles of life.

There is a saying in Ayurveda that says "the mind follows the body and the body follows the mind," meaning that whatever we put into our sensory perceptions will eventually affect the mind and then eventually lead to how we live our life and how our atma (or soul) is ultimately nourished.

When it comes to the bodywork portion of Ayurveda, it is indeed an art form. Getting issues out of our tissues is done with ease with treatments that lull the mind, body, and spirit to a deep subtle state of consciousness. In this state, we're able to connect with our inner intelligence, allowing the channels (called srotas) to open up, allowing the issues to flow properly in order for them to be digested or expelled out.

The bodywork practitioner must be in tune with the basics of Ayurveda and its fundamental knowledge in order to be able to be as clear in their own perceptions and have an inner quality of peacefulness (known as sattva) in order to convey the Ayurvedic vidya properly. It is an inherent intuition that allows prana to flow from the healer's hands to the receiver. This quality is pure love. Besides the love that flows from one being to another, in Ayurveda oil (or snehna) means love. And as massage therapists, we all know that besides technique, love is the single most influential modality used in healing. When a practitioner comes from love through their heart then a deep sense of nourishment occurs within the tissues. This is healing in a nutshell!

When the body is settled and relaxes into total bliss, the body channels open up, allowing the healing process to occur; by the way this also happens during meditation. These are just some of the techniques that are done on a daily basis in an Ayurvedic lifestyle and through Ayurvedic bodywork. Yes, the practitioners are actually in a meditative state when they practice… Well, hopefully they are. It's within this state of consciousness where the body has the permission to maintain homeostasis and hence re-enliven its baseline consciousness to achieve true harmony and balance with nature, provided the diet and lifestyle are also balanced. When all of these factors are in line with the individual's base line constitution, issues have a hard time sticking anywhere within the consciousness of the individual. Issues easily digest, resolve, let go, and become our daily nourishment.

As part of our daily maintenance of our systems, we do a daily (sometimes twice daily) oil massage in specific patterns on the body, which helps support circulation of blood and lymph that nourish and relax the entire system, including the nervous system. This is called a basic abhyanga. Most everyone can enjoy it, but it should still ideally be under the advisement of an Ayurvedic practitioner, or even doctor in some cases, if an individual wanted to go deeper within understanding true Ayurveda. Under the watchful eye of the practitioner, they will determine your exact needs by assessing your basic constitution, age, stage in which the disease has manifested, your state of agni (digestion), the aggravated dosha (elemental qualities) that needs to be brought back into balance, and determine if ama (undigested physical and mental stuff) is present within your system. All of these factors will then determine which types of Ayurvedic chikitsa will be right for you (there are many different modalities), as well as what type and how much oil to use and when.

On a larger, more detoxing scale these processes are more in depth in preparation (purvakarma) for panchakarma (PK), which is a major phase of purification that helps stop and even reverse the disease process within the body. PK cleanses and purifies the whole system, which includes all seven dhatus (physiological tissues) while building up and restoring the agni (digestive fire) as the foundation in Ayurveda. Within this the practitioner is considering time or age of client or season; space; and a proper diet of fresh, seasonal, and nourishing foods. Treatments such as herbal supplementation, meditation, yoga, more massage, and a shift in the diet and lifestyle are gentle, nourishing, and critical in the restoration of the body's natural systems.

True Ayurveda is not a cookie-cutter solution to any one issue within our tissues but it is a way of life based on mindfulness practices and gentle guidance of an experienced Ayurvedic practitioner to help you navigate what your system is and what it needs. It's kind of like having a good mechanic for your car. At best, Ayurveda prevents issues from sticking within our tissues. Even better, Ayurveda has the ability (in some cases) to reverse the disease process by bringing the natural elements back into balance; things that one might have brought out of balances through overuse or underuse and misuse of the senses.

When the appropriate treatment is properly administered at the right time, with the right oils, and the right intention, I have personally seen these Ayurvedic treatments and procedures help many people find relief from diseases such as fibromyalgia, Parkinson's, rheumatoid arthritis, obesity, mental disorders, constipation, skin disorders, and general stress, just to name a few. It brings me great joy to witness the transformation not only within the physical body of the individual but the mind and spirit as well. The treatments are still very powerful on their own if one plans on doing them on a daily, weekly, or even biweekly occurrence. It is then advised that one should be under the guidance of a highly qualified practitioner of Ayurveda or doctor of Ayurveda. Do your research when finding the proper practitioner for you. Check their references and schools. A one-year crash course in Ayurveda is not generally enough to guide you through purvakarma, panchakarma, and paschatkarma. You want a seasoned professional for this kind of detox, but the holistic health counselor can guide you on the right path through proper diet and lifestyle and start your journey to health and wellness.

So in a nutshell, our balanced well-being, free of disease or "issues within our tissues" relies upon our proper choices in diet, lifestyle, and knowledge. The lack of proper knowledge of these or misuse of senses sets the groundwork for disease to become lodged within our tissues. Rather than using a one-size-fits-all approach, Ayurveda uses an extremely personalized approach to healing. Treatments and medicines are prescribed based on an individual's needs with regard to their lifestyle. Although Ayurveda takes symptomatology into account, its focus is on the process and not on the symptom; symptoms are the clues. Ayurveda is not a one pill wonder or one massage wonder. It is, however, an ever-expanding awareness that has the ability to create balance and give us the biggest defense in warding off disease and issues. Ayurveda is a force that has been emerging for centuries based upon Vedic wisdom brought down from the heavens to help us live a balanced and harmonious life on this planet.

Tapping Technique

I asked renowned tapping technique instructor and author Alina Frank to explain to us what Emotional Freedom Technique/Tapping Technique is and how it can help us heal. I also asked her to give us instruction on how to treat ourselves. Here is her offering:

EFT Explained by Alina Frank

There is a healing modality growing in popularity and usage around the world that is known as the emotional freedom techniques (EFT) and commonly referred to as "tapping." Individuals are finding this approach to be both quick and effective in reducing suffering related to physical pain and discomfort. Tapping is used as a powerful self-help tool as well as being utilized by counseling and healing arts professionals, life coaches, and peak performance experts throughout the world. EFT directly targets both the body's physiological stress response along with reducing the negative emotions, such as frustration and disappointment, that coincide with painful physical conditions. By providing a great sense of control over stress-influenced pain, a concurrent reduction in the stress-response ensues, offering even further relief from symptoms. Tapping is swiftly growing in public acceptance, media mentions, and peer-reviewed research. Enthusiastic proponents have included Drs. Bruce Lipton, Candace Pert, Deepak Chopra, Norm Shealy, Wayne Dyer, and many more respected professionals that are leaders in body-mind approaches to health.

Stress and Health

The body's immediate response to an event that feels dangerous or threatening is a natural and useful one to keep us safe and alive. Some situations that are not truly threatening to our physical survival can elicit the very same stress response in our bodies as a truly dangerous one. When a vehicle suddenly stops short in front of you on the highway, it is appropriate for your body to engage in a life-preserving physical reaction. However, it is not appropriate to have that same reaction when you receive a memo from your boss. When this kind of response happens on a regular basis with work, in family relationships, or with regards to your finances, the effect can be extremely detrimental.

Cumulative stress-inducing events such as these have an additive effect over time and have been shown to have significantly harmful effects on your health. The "stress response," as originally described by Hans Selye, MD, and supported by current research, is a multipronged reaction that combines an elevation of stress hormones, such as epinephrine and cortisol, as well as emotional and psychological reactions. Sustained levels of such stress hormones have been associated with increased biological aging, impairment of brain function and structure, decreased immune response, deterioration of many health conditions including heart disease and cancer as well as increased incidence of chronic pain.

Stress, Negative Emotions, and EFT

Just as there are appropriate levels of stress, there are also appropriate levels of emotional expression. It is alright to feel scared when your company suddenly announces upcoming layoffs. When you are betrayed by your spouse, anger would be a normal response. If, however, your fear and anger ruminate in your mind for years or hibernate within your subconscious, then this too can be harmful. Your negative life experiences have either been healed and integrated into your life's wisdom or they can be stuck and prevent your growth and development. When you can't overcome a negative life experience and avoid dealing with it and perhaps suppress the emotions associated with it, your body may well become the messenger for what has not been expressed. With EFT, you work with the messenger and uncover the hidden metaphors in order to heal. For example, a sharp pain between your shoulder blades could signify a betrayal—literally the feeling of having been stabbed in the back.

In traditional Chinese medicine, "chi" (or vital life force energy) flows freely through channels referred to as meridians. Negative emotions and traumas can block this flow. EFT utilizes and stimulates these acupoints on the face and upper body that are close to the surface of the skin so that needles are not required. By physically tapping on these points while simultaneously reciting specific statements acknowledging how you feel about a certain stressful situation, the blockage dissipates, allowing your body to heal itself. One common description of EFT refers to the technique as emotional acupuncture without needles.

There are currently more than sixty peer-reviewed research papers that report clinical outcomes using EFT with over 90 percent of them demonstrating its effectiveness. They have shown statistically significant reductions in pain (i.e., fibromyalgia, tension headaches), stress hormone levels, anxiety, phobias, and post-traumatic stress, as well as the enhancement of athletic performance and even the reduction of food cravings with ensuing weight loss.

—Alina Frank and Craig Weiner, DC, EFT Tapping Master Trainers
www.efttappingtraining.com

The Acupoints

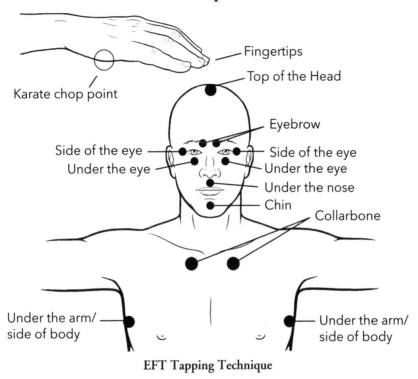

EFT Tapping Technique

I also asked Alina Frank to teach us how to do a self-treatment. This is her offering to us:

Tapping FAQ by Alina Frank

For starters, let's go over the acupoints that we use in EFT. There are hundreds of acupoints all over your body, but when tapping, we focus on the nine described below. You can activate these easily by tapping them yourself. Here are descriptions of acupoint locations in the order in which you'll tap them.

1. Side of Hand (SH): The outer edge of your palm, between the base of your little finger and wrist.

2. Eyebrow (EB): On the inside of your eyebrow, right where your eyebrow begins.

3. Side of Eye (SE): On the bony ridge between your eye and your temple. Be gentle with this point. It's a sensitive spot for some people.

4. Under Eye (UE): On the bone under your eye, in line with your pupil.

5. Under Nose (UN): Centered between the bottom of the nose and the top of the upper lip.

6. Chin (CH): Centered between the bottom of the lower lip and the chin.

7. Collarbone (CB): Locate the U-shaped dip at the top of your sternum (under your Adam's apple), then move down your body an inch and to either side an inch. Because this point is significant, I suggest that you activate both sides at once by making a fist with one hand (to create a larger surface) and gently thump the area where a man would tie a necktie.

8. Under Arm (UA): About four inches beneath your armpit, where a woman's bra band passes as it wraps around her rib cage.

9. Top of Head (TH): The very top of your head. If you imagine that you're a marionette and the top of your head is attached to a cord, you'll easily locate this point.

How quickly should I tap?

The rate at which you tap is quick, but not rushed. Find a free metronome online (for example, visit a.bestmetronome.com) and set it to 240 beats per minute. That's about right, but it's also okay to go slower, especially as you're learning.

How often should I tap each point?

You'll tap your SH point continually as you say your setup statement three times. (These statements are personal, and there is not room to expand on them here.) You'll tap each of the remaining acupoints while saying your reminder phrase at each point—tapping approximately three to seven times. (Some reminder phrases are longer than others, so you wind up tapping more often when you say those.)

How much pressure should I use?

Drum your fingertips on a table or desktop. That's about how hard to tap. Harder is not better.

How important is it to tap the exact location of the acupoint?

Just try to get as close as you can. When you tap, the vibration affects a larger area and is usually enough to activate the point without your needing to be exactly on it.

Does it matter which hand I use?

You can use either or both hands. It's usually more comfortable to use your dominant hand to tap your nondominant side.

Flower Remedies

Pamela Bellamy, L.A.c., is my acupuncturist, Reiki teacher, spiritual teacher, and very dear friend. I chose to interview her on flower remedies. One of the more widely known flower remedies that you may have heard is Bach's Rescue Remedy, which is used to calm the nervous system. There are other flower essences that are also used for specific needs as well. According to Pamela, "The flower essences do not treat illness, they treat emotions."

In her practice she uses needles, herbs, energy healing, and flower remedies as needed. She says that emotions are a key way to distort the physical body noted within the organ systems. Using the five elements in Chinese medicine, the organ system belongs to each element and the corresponding emotions. If someone were displaying weakness in one of the elements, she believes those to be long-standing emotional imbalances. She will then muscle test (muscle testing/applied kinesiology will be described in the glossary) and compare it to the organ system that appears most imbalanced.

From there she may blend a flower essence formula (no more than six essences in a blend is her personal blending preference) to help the person lift the layers of those particular emotions. She said that emotions are like an onion, you can peel back layer by layer or you can cut it in half and get right to the heart of it depending on the blends that you create and for which purpose. In her description of the essences, you don't have to necessarily revisit the traumas, but this is more to help lift off the layers of the emotions that have been built up from something recent or something you've spent a lifetime holding down.

Chinese Medicine and Acupuncture

Chinese Medicine includes herbal medicine, acupuncture, dietary therapy, exercise such as tai chi and qigong, massage (tui na). Chinese medicine utilizes many techniques, such

such as acupuncture, to heal the body. I will share my own little story to let you know that acupuncture can treat many things that in our culture are considered "idiopathic," meaning it does not have a definitive cause or cure. My acupuncturist, Pamela, treated and cleared a friend's Bell's palsy in two sessions. Bell's palsy is a paralysis of one side of the face. In the West, we have no understanding or standard treatment for it. That friend referred me to my acupuncturist for my own problem.

At the time, I was dealing with a really traumatic problem with hives. I went to an allergist from Harvard who actually said, "Whatever your problem is, allergies ain't it." She did all sorts of tests on me and to no avail. I was stuck on medication for allergies for nine months when I was not actually allergic to anything known. I went to Pamela for the first time for something entirely different. I mentioned to her that I was on a medication for hives but that I had not taken it that day in case it would interfere with our treatment. She looked completely unphased and said, "Well, let's go ahead and clear that up, and then we can focus on the thing that you came for." I thought, *Okay, yeah right...let's just clear that up. I'm sure it's that easy. That's why I've been going from doctor to doctor and put on medicine because it's just that simple.* Well...I can honestly say that this was more than twelve years ago and I have never taken that allergy medicine ever again, nor ever dealt with a single issue of hives ever since that day. That is huge. That was life changing for me and to her it was something very simple and treatable. That is Chinese medicine. Things that you are unable to figure out or find answers to in allopathic medicine might be very simply defined and treatable with acupuncture.

Meridians

One of the basic tenets of traditional Chinese medicine holds that the body's vital energy (chi or qi) circulates through channels, called meridians, that have branches connected to bodily organs and functions. As discussed briefly in chapter 2, meridians are the energy lines that flow along the matrix of the fascia in the body. Each meridian is a channel from a specific organ in the body. The organs according to Chinese medicine all have high and low emotions that correspond to the actual function of the organ itself. Each organ also has cravings of food types and times of day where they are strongest and weakest. There is so much information on meridians that we could get lost introducing basics. In this chart, I narrowed it down to the meridian itself, whether it is yin (feminine) or yang (masculine), what organ/meridian is the pair to it and the emotions when out of balance. I did not go into detail on when in balance, as they are simply the opposite of what is out of balance. An example is when a person is fearful and unsure, the balanced version would be confident and steady.

Yin Meridian	Yang Meridian
Lung Meridian: Controls breath and energy. Energy commands the blood. If energy flows, blood flows. **Emotions out of balance:** Sadness, grief, anxiety, shame.	**Large Intestine Meridian:** Controls the waste onward to excretion. Helps to balance body fluids. **Emotions out of balance:** Worry, sadness, grief. Fears can cause the nervous poopies.
Spleen Meridian: (This meridian includes the pancreas in Chinese Medicine): Controls extraction of nutrients, regulates how much and how well the blood circulates. Works with kidneys both energetically and physically for fluid balance. Emotionally the spleen channel helps with analytical thinking, intelligence, memory. **Emotions out of balance:** Excessive thinking, obsessive thoughts, regret, doubt.	**Stomach Meridian:** This is our place of nourishment. Digests fluids and solid foods. **Emotions out of balance:** Severe anxiety, mental imbalances, mania.
Heart Meridian: This is the king organ and houses the spirit. **Emotions out of balance:** Hate, guilt, craves external things.	**Small Intestine:** Once food leaves the stomach, the small intestine helps further digest and refine the food—it separates what is to be kept and what is to be released. **Emotions out of balance:** Mental clarity can be compromised, insecurity, restless thinking patterns, wishy-washy in decisions.

Yin Meridian	Yang Meridian
Kidney Meridian (Also includes the adrenal glands since they sit on top of the kidneys): Kidneys filter fluid and release fluids. Adrenals secrete hormones that govern metabolism, sexual potency, and more. These areas govern our place of will power. **Emotions out of balance:** Fearful, insecure, feeling isolated from the outside world.	**Bladder Meridian:** Stores and excretes waste from the body through the urine. **Emotions out of balance:** This area governs anger issues. When you are pissed…you are literally pissed off. The bladder feels it, controls it, and suppresses it all. Grudges live here. Jealousy and suspicious actions live in this house.
Pericardium Meridian: The pericardium is the sack around the heart that protects it. When a practitioner sees an issue with the pericardium channel, they send you to a cardiologist. When they see an issue with the heart channel, they send you to a psychologist. **Emotions out of balance:** Phobic behavior lives in this house. Difficulties with being honest with your emotions come from this space.	**Triple Warmer Meridian:** This is an energy that is not even recognized in the West. It oversees activity within all the other organs. It helps with circulation and the nourishment of all circulatory energies within the body. It regulates the body's fluids as a general statement. **Emotions out of balance:** This is the place where a sexual overdrive can occur. It can burn out the body and lead to serious consequences of burnout of the other organs. It can wreak havoc among the reproductive organs.

Yin Meridian	Yang Meridian
Liver Meridian: Detoxifies the body fluids. Stores the blood, replenishes the blood and fluids (blood, plasma, proteins, etc.). The liver governs the amount of blood glucose and so much more. **Emotions out of balance:** The liver is known for its ability to have rage and anger issues. Resentments, jealousy, and depression all store in this house.	**Gallbladder Meridian:** Secrets bile fluid that help digest and metabolize in the body. Works directly with the liver both physically and emotionally. **Emotions out of balance:** The liver/gallbladder run along the lines between the eyebrows. A person who carries a lot of aggression has deep lines in this space. This is an energy of extreme anger, frustration, and nonmovement when at the high load of the out of balance energy.
Conception Vessel: These two meridians form a full circle of energy from the front to the back of the body. The conception vessel nourishes all the yin channels in the body.	**Governing Vessel:** Nourishes all the yang vessels in the body.
* It is believed that when doing energy work, placing the tip of the tongue against the roof of the mouth at the small mountain just behind the two front teeth connect these two vessels together, allowing the energy to circulate through your body only leaving through your hands. It is practiced during attunements to energy work and other avenues of healing to gain clarity and gather the strength of the energy being produced.	

Introduction to Meditation: Seated Practice Contextualized

Stephen Watson was mentioned in the introduction in regard to meditation. Below are his simplified techniques that he offers in his classes. The reason that I reached out to Stephen for this information is that he teaches meditation all over the world. He has simplified it in such a way that it can help us get out of the mind struggles and loops that we have so often when confronting stillness. Here is his offering on meditation practice:

A Brief Sitting Practice by Stephen Watson

The following well-worn and life-tested instructions are designed to be simple yet comprehensive while requiring no introduction or commentary:

> See to your discomforts.
> See to your comforts.
> Become comfortable with any/all remaining discomforts.
> Practice.
> Welcome back the discomforts.
> Return to the mundane world.

See? You already got it. Seeing as this is a book, I'll add some commentary now. But the commentary won't help you understand or get this framework for practice, it will simply deepen it. I've taught hundreds of students with no preamble, just a line by line reading of the above. You already got it!

Sitting Practice, Contextualized

See to your discomforts. Remove what will detract from your practice. Address those things that are pressing/painful/distracting or that will otherwise challenge your practice. Within each aspect of self (psychological, physical, mental, emotional, etc.), see to the first thing on the list of discomforts there.

See to your comforts. Add what will add to your practice. Address those things that are not painful/distracting or that will otherwise challenge your practice but which, if addressed, will improve your practice or your ability to engage in your practice. Within each aspect of self (psychological, physical, mental, emotional, etc.), see to the first thing on the list of comforts there. Same durations? Do you detect an urge to spend more time on one than the other?

Become comfortable with any/all remaining discomforts. This does not mean to ignore/distract from/push aside those discomforts.

Practice. Sit.

Welcome back the discomforts. Whether you recognize them or they are new. Whether or not they recognize you. Do not see to the discomforts; to sincerely welcome something is to invite and greet it, as it is. There is no preference for one's guest to change, dissolve, or exit.

Forgiveness

Forgiveness for many of us is a concept that is particularly difficult to put into motion. I hope that this guidance does help you on your journey.

A Practice on Forgiveness: A Continuation on Forgiveness by Ashli Callaway

Forgiveness is a learned skill that must be practiced consistently in order to maintain proficiency or pursue mastery. Some people have more of a natural proclivity for it than others, but anyone willing to practice can learn to play. To prepare for this practice, write down a list of the people you want to forgive. Don't skip the writing part—it is essential to the process.

Write beside each of those people a bullet list of the facts you want to forgive them for. No judgments—only facts. Examples of judgments would be "he betrayed me," "she broke my heart," or "he ruined my life."

Next write any feeling you have that does not feel good can be categorized as either anger, fear, or sadness, so choose one of the three that most accurately reflects how you felt when the fact happened and how you feel about it now. If you are not sure, reflect on where you feel the memory in your body, and work back from there to the feeling.

Beside each feeling, write what rule or boundary of yours was broken. You might think you don't have rules, but you do. Own them—even if they are ugly—and write them down. Finally, rank your list from highest to lowest in terms of investment of your time, energy, and emotions—most painful to least painful.

Now that you have outlined and organized who and what you are wanting to forgive, you need a working definition of forgiveness. Carolyn Myss says in her book *Anatomy of the Spirit*:

> *Forgiveness is not the same as telling the person who harmed you, "it's okay," which is more or less the way most people view it. Rather, forgiveness is a complex act of consciousness... that liberates the psyche and soul from the need for personal vengeance and the perception of oneself as a victim. More than releasing from blame the people*

who caused our wounds, it means releasing the control that the perception of victim-hood has over our psyche.[4]

Find a definition that feels liberating to you, and use it in your practice so you are clear with yourself what you want the outcome to be. Write the definition you choose at the top of your paper.

Now you have almost everything you need to practice forgiveness in front of you and in the heart of who you are. If you need some time or distance from this before you go any further, take it. When you are ready, the rest—like the game Othello—takes a minute to learn and a lifetime to master. And, two minutes of practice a day.

Look at the bottom of your list. Read what you wrote there—name, facts, feelings, rules. And, ask yourself this question: **Just for today, am I willing to forgive _____?**

Be deeply honest with yourself and trust your answer—yes or no. Either answer, truthfully and lovingly given, is the right one. If, for today, the answer is no, then love yourself and look back at the feelings you wrote beside the facts—anger, fear, or sadness.

If you wrote *anger*, then your practice today is to sit quietly for two minutes, breathing deeply, and say to yourself with your inhale: **I love myself**, and with your exhale: **I give up my craving for power and control.**

If you wrote *fear*, then your practice today is to sit quietly for two minutes, breathing deeply, and say to yourself with your inhale: **I love myself**, and with your exhale: **I give up my craving for security and survival.**

If you wrote *sadness*, then your practice today is to sit quietly for two minutes, breathing deeply, and say to yourself with your inhale: **I love myself**, and with your exhale: **I give up my craving for affection and approval.**

If tomorrow the answer is still no, love yourself and your no, and repeat the practice daily until the answer is yes. If, for today, the answer is yes, then your practice is to pray for the other person's happiness. You will likely find you are unable to compose a prayer for the happiness of someone who hurt you, so I've included the prayer I use in my own forgiveness practice that you are welcome to.

---

4. Carolyn Myss, *Anatomy of the Spirit* (New York: Three Rivers Press, 1996), 215.

May I be peaceful, happy, and healthy in body, mind, and spirit.

May I be safe and free from harm.

May I be free from any attachments to anger, fear, and sadness.

May _____ be peaceful, happy, and healthy in body, mind, and spirit.

May _____ be safe and free from harm.

May _____ be free from any attachments to anger, fear, and sadness.

May everybody be peaceful, happy, and healthy in body, mind, and spirit.

May everybody be safe and free from harm.

May everybody be free from any attachments to anger, fear, and sadness.[5]

Whether you use this prayer or a short one of your own, write it on the bottom of your paper so you can see it whenever you sit to practice. Breathe deeply, read or recite the prayer, and when two minutes have passed your practice is over. Whether you are working with yes or with no, when two minutes have passed, let it go for the rest of the day. No matter how many times or how intensely your desire to wrestle with it comes up, gently, patiently, and persistently put it down like you would a new puppy determined to climb up your pants leg, and do not pick it up again until tomorrow.

When you follow these instructions consistently with a commitment to loving yourself and even a little bit of hope, you will find that in just a little while you will experience forgiveness in a very real and powerful way.

Toe Reading

When I interviewed Cheryl Speen on the toe reading and map of the feet and hands, I was fascinated with what she had to say. She teaches a full course on this subject at the Southwest Institute of Healing Arts. She can actually see trauma that has occurred in one's body by the lines on the feet. While she cannot teach such detailed information in this offering, if you find yourself curious to know more, please look into this course to help you. Here is her offering on the feet and toes:

---

5. Thich Nhat Hahn, *Teachings on Love* (Berkeley, CA: Parallax Press, 1998), 21.

Toe Reading by Cheryl Speen

If the mind is not ready to witness/accept what the body went through, then the body will not mark it—you will not pick it up. The body completely covers it until the mind is ready to witness it. Our ankles represent our pleasure zone. All of the reproductive organs show up around the ankles. This could be lack of pleasure in all aspects of our lives, not just sexual or physical. Broken ankles may represent not taking the time to have fun, working too much, or not taking a break until spirit decides you need one.

Our feet are our foundation. Everything in our life rests on our feet. Although our hips and legs are the momentum that moves us forward, our feet have the power to stop or start any progress or process. Swellings, pain, or numbness in the feet could all be factors of not connecting with the earth beneath you—the earth that supports and sustains you.

Toes, fingers, and ears are about the details of life. The feet represent our past, the hands are the present moment, and the ears are about a propensity of the future. Understanding those three aspects of the extremities can help determine what the details may entail.

In reflexology, the feet play a major role in recognizing the stories that are showing up throughout the entire body. Starting at the toes, you can work your way down the foot from head to toe witnessing markings, colorings, changes in texture in the feet based on the areas they are showing up.

The toes are where the head and neck are depicted. The balls of the feet are the chest, heart, and lungs. The upper arch shows the start of the digestive area with the stomach/spleen/pancreas and the liver/gallbladder, the lower arch shows the middle digestive—small intestine, ileocecal valve, appendix—and the end of the digestive process—large intestine. The heel has the hips, legs, and feet.

Looking at the foot from the top to bottom, you can also see how the body can show up from big toe to small toe. Big toe is the head. The second toe is the chest/breast, the third toe is the upper digestive area. The fourth toe is the lower digestive area, and lastly the fifth toe represents the hips, leg, and feet.

Since the toes/fingers and ears represent the details in our life—we can go much deeper into the meanings of what may be taking place in the mental/emotional world.

The fingers will show things that are happening in the now, but since the now is just a minute flash in time, unless there is a chronic problem, it probably will not be as easily seen as in the toes. This makes witnessing the stories in the toes much easier to see, so I will use the toes as my base.

Each toe is an element. The big toe is the ether, second toe is air, third toe is fire, fourth toe is water, and fifth toe is earth.

When describing the elements of each toe, you can witness what might be happening in someone's life. Although we never know for sure, asking questions rather than stating what you see will help someone witness what they might subconsciously be holding back. Bringing it into the present moment can illicit a lot of *aha* moments and help someone overcome self-sabotaging thinking that they may have created a habit of from early years and not even realize what they have been subconsciously creating.

The ether is about the space within the space—everything in life is connected in one way or another and the space of ether is that connection. If you think in terms of the Big Bang Theory, everything was created from no thing and that no thing is ether. I like to think of this space as the Space of Infinite Possibility. So if the big toe is the head and the head is where all of thoughts, ideas, and beliefs come from, then this is the Place of Infinite Possibility. Our thoughts begin here, who we are and, since ether encompasses all the other elements—so the head governs all the other aspects of the body—we like to call this toe, the destiny toe.

Appendix C

Collective Responses from a Survey of Other Health and Bodywork Professionals

I asked a respected professor and psychologist who teaches field research at a university to help me to create a survey. My intention was to interview as many people in the health-care industry as possible at the start of this book. I wanted to see how many people had the same information that I do in regard to the muscles and emotions. I had more than fifty people respond and fill out the survey. Below is a compilation of answers.

Q: What is your training and specialty?

A: These are the combined professions that participated in this survey: massage therapist (deep tissue), acupressure, Ayurvedic bodywork, energy work, energy system education, holistic therapeutic, foot reflexology, nurturing therapeutic massage, health promotion, education, and behavior (DrPH) associate of applied science in medical kinesio taping, medical massage therapy, chiropractor, emergency management, connective tissue massage, Reiki, polarity therapy, shamanic healing, traditional Chinese medicine, integrative wellness, auriculotherapy (ear), master of acupuncture and Oriental medicine, massage & bodywork therapist, Qi Gong & martial arts instructor, nurse massage therapist (RN, LMT), sports massage therapy, body movement (dance), core myofascial release, Rossiter coach, neuro reflex release, Quantum Touch Energetics, ortho manual therapy, integrated bodywork, NRT work, Swedish massage, shiatsu, structural/postural analysis, myofascial, lymphatic drainage, speciality Thai healing methods, orthopedic massage, prenatal focus, osteopathic family physician. 1500+ hours Training in the United States and Thailand...

Q: Do you associate emotions with particular muscles or areas in the body?
A: Yes was 69.77 percent of all responders.
No was 30.23 percent of all responders.

Q: What are your thoughts on emotions being stored in the body?
A: The answers ranged from absolutely undeniable to I don't know. Some answers were extremely specific, backing up their belief that emotions are in fact stored in the body while others were more optimistic but don't know for sure.

Q: How did you learn that particular muscles are associated with emotions?
A: The answers ranged from massage, acupuncture, any extensive schooling to personal experience.

Q: What emotions have you found in the neck (posterior) and neck (anterior)?
A: The answers were fairly wide ranging from stress patterns, anxiety, lack of flexibility in their daily lives both physically and mentally, rigid behaviors, fearful behaviors.

Q: What emotions have you found in the mouth, jaw, or face?
A: Most responses here were focused on anger, stress, holding on to things, and lack of flexibility.

Q: What emotions have you found in the arms, forearms, or wrists?
A: Heart patterns in the feminine energy, rigid behaviors around the wrists, grief, and fear were the common threads of these responses.

Q: What emotions have you found in the legs, hips, hip flexors, or glutes?
A: The answers here went from anger to fear to holding on to the past to procrastination patterns. Fear of the future, disconnectedness, loneliness, and resistance to moving forward were answers here as well.

Q: What emotions have you found in the trunk or vital organs?

A: These answers seem to focus on trust, love, forgiveness, sense of self or not feeling a true sense of self, love or loss of love, vulnerable feelings, worry, grief, fear. Anger, joy, anticipation, decision-making, or being indecisive lives in this space as well.

Q: What emotions have you found in the hands or feet?

A: The answers here focused on genetic lines of emotion, patterns of karma, self-expectancy, life, love, stress, worry, fear, compassion, truth. Also a focus around giving and receiving from this space.

Q: What emotions have you found in the shoulders or back?

A: Letting go of the past, betrayal, each vertebrae is a different energy, bracing and embracing, ego, feeling the weight of the world, feeling responsible, stress, burdens, worry, carrying old baggage, sadness, stress, and fear.

Q: What emotions have you found in the chest?

A: The overall consensus was joy, love, compassion, vulnerability, confirmations from spirit, sorrow, guilt, love/hate, holding on too tight to something, pain, despair, fear, hope, sadness.

Q: How do you treat emotions in the body? What do you treat?

A: Because so many people work in different avenues of health care the answers to this question were very specific to their practice. The people overall work slowly and treat the person by meeting them where they are and gently guiding the body to release old patterns and pains. This is done by energy work, regulating their breathing, needling, herbs, heat, holding the space for them, massage, aromatherapy, adding pillows in for them to hold on to or cry into.

Glossary

I will introduce this glossary with a quick story. I worked on a client once who had hardened circles in the middle of her tendon along the bottoms of her feet. It was the same on both feet. I felt them and asked right away what they were. She replied with "they are fallen tendons." After I sat with this explanation, I probed a little deeper: "Who diagnosed this? Did you see a podiatrist?" She said to me that she had no idea what a podiatrist was and that her general practitioner suggested that could be what it was. I asked her to please go home and make an appointment with the podiatrist (a foot doctor).

I say this to emphasize that it is important that people know where to look when there are issues in their bodies. Listed below is a detailed compilation of every healing modality mentioned in this book and beyond. Some people will be inspired to find a shaman; others may need something more physical like a rolfing practitioner. Also included is a list of terms that apply to these types of work. I hope that this detailed glossary provides some insight to such questions.

Abduction—Movement away from the centerline of the body.

Acupressure—Refers to any number of treatment systems that manipulate acupoints. Philosophy comes from traditional Chinese acupuncture. Includes touching, pressing, or rubbing pressure points. Does not use needles or herbs.

Acupuncture—Chinese medicine. Works with the whole body, mind, and spirit. It is used with needles and herbs to treat the whole person. Many times when Western medicine can't treat something effectively, acupuncture can. This can address so many different ailments it's difficult to put into one category. Can help with serious illness, pain, autoimmune disorders, nausea, infertility, and much more. It works with the body's meridians.

Adduction—Movement toward the centerline of the body.

Alexander Technique—Movement education to relearn postural and eighty-nine movement habits.

Antagonist—Muscle that is exactly opposite of the primary muscle.

Applied Kinesiology—A series of muscle tests in which the muscles test strong or weak depending on the circumstance. This can provide detailed insight into the subconscious body and mind for available treatments.

Ashiatsu—Used with the feet. The therapist holds on to bars on the ceiling and is able to deliver a lot of pressure with their feet.

Chi/Ki/Prana—In the United States, we do not have a word describing this. Chi is Chinese. Ki is Japanese, and Prana is Hindu/Yoga. It all refers to the same life force energy.

Cognitive Therapy/Cognitive Behavioral Therapy—Talk therapy. This works with how the mind reacts to situations and helps assist in creating more effective behavior patterns.

Chiropractic—Stresses the body's natural recuperative abilities. Emphasis is on the alignment of the spinal column and its effect on the nervous system.

CranioSacral Therapy—Developed by osteopathic physician John E. Upledger. A gentle, hands-on method of evaluating and enhancing the functioning of the cranial sacral system—comprised of the membranes and cerebrospinal fluid that surround and protect the brain and spinal cord. Is wonderful for emotional trauma as well.

Distal—Farther from the point of attachment.

Dorsiflex—Toes pulling up toward the face away from the floor.

Fascia—Strong connective tissue covering muscle bundles.

Feldenkrais Method—Somatic education using awareness through movement and functional integration.

Healing Touch^{TM}—This is referred to as energy therapy. The practitioner uses their hands consciously to help support the body for physical, emotional, spiritual, and mental health. It is believed they can influence the magnetic field around the body with their hands. This is a heart-based practice and is widely accepted in hospitals and other healing facilities.

Hot Stone Therapy—This massage includes heated rocks either laid along the body or used in the hands of the practitioner to deliver a deeper relaxation response through the heat.

Hypnotherapy—Can allow you to escape from typical responses and behaviors that are not in your best interest by using light hypnosis. Know that when you go for hypnotherapy, you are still conscious. You do know what is going on around you. It is a way of reprogramming the responses to habits. It is commonly used for cessation of smoking, weight loss, and release of trauma.

Inferior—Lower body.

Insertion—Where the muscle attaches.

Integrative Medicine—Treat the whole person approach to health. This medicine combines complementary medicine such as yoga, tai chi, acupuncture, herbs, massage, biofeedback.

Lateral—Wide from the center.

Lomi Lomi Massage—This massage technique is native to Hawaii. It is a smooth massage likened to cat paws that work out the muscles and relax the body. *Lomi Lomi* translates to the words "knead" or "smooth."

Manual Lymph Drainage—Developed by Dr. Emile Vodder is a series of gentle, rhythmic movements to move proteins and tissue fluid to lymph nodes that are fully functioning. This is used for sinus issues, swelling, sprains, strains, and lymphedema. Also for pre/post-surgery to reduce swelling, bruising, and scarring.

Massage Therapy—Manual soft tissue manipulation to positively affect the body. Massage has two main types of effect: mechanical effects, direct physical effect on the tissues treated, and reflex effects, indirect effect on the body functions and tissues through the response of the nervous or energy systems of the body.

Medial—Center or midline.

Meridian—There are twelve channels of chi. These correspond to the main organs in the body.

Myofascial Release—This is a massage technique that treats immobilized skeletal muscles. It is a hands-on manipulation to relax contracted muscles. This style works directly with the fascia.

Nambudripad's Allergy Elimination Technique (NAET)—Uses applied kinesiology (*see separate entry*) to test sensitivities and treat them.

Naturopath—Based on the body's ability to heal itself. Naturopaths use modalities such as herbs, homeopathy, acupuncture, massage, hydrotherapy, nutrition, and exercise.

Neuromuscular Therapy—Soft tissue manipulation involving ischemic compression on or near trigger points, gliding thumb strokes, skin rolling, and stretching movements. A trigger point is noted when there is referring pain—meaning that when a certain muscle or soft tissue has pressure applied, there is pain radiating to another part of the body.

Occupational Therapy—Occupational therapy is specific to a population that has sustained an injury or was born with certain inhabiting qualities that limit movement in daily life. Its function is to teach or reteach tasks to achieve independence and a better quality of life.

Origin—Where the muscle starts.

Orthopedic Massage—Involves treatment of soft tissues with manipulation and assessment to reduce dysfunction of the skeletal muscles and fascia. This massage style helps restore structural balance and minimize pain.

Orthopedic Medicine—Specializes in the treatment of joints, bones, and muscular system. Usually associated with sports medicine.

Osteopath—Emphasizes the body's ability to heal itself. Stresses proper functioning of the body's nervous system and musculoskeletal systems as well as the body's fluid systems to flow properly. Fully licensed to diagnose, prescribe drugs, and perform surgery.

Panchakarma—A detoxification process from Ayurvedic medicine that involves herbal therapy, massage, and other therapies to help the body release toxins and maintain balanced health.

Physical Therapy—Deals with a wide range of conditions. Uses physical medicine techniques—exercise, myofascial release/massage, hydrotherapy (water-ice/heat), ultrasound, joint mobilization. Works with post-operative cases, neurological conditions, stroke and paralysis cases, and more. I like this work the best for post-injury operations.

Physiology—Anatomy in motion. A physiologist tests your body on the various physiological processes including cardiac, exercise, and respiratory physiology.

Physiotherapy—Also referred to as physical therapy is within conventional medicine. It is basically the same thing as physical therapy and generally practiced only by physical therapists. In some states, it is associated with a doctorate of physical therapy.

Plantar Flex—Pointing toes down toward the floor.

Podiatrist—Deals with issues in the feet and lower extremity.

Polarity Therapy—Developed by Randolph Stone, naturopath, chiropractor, and osteopath. Combines both Eastern and Western practices. Includes diet, exercise, and thinking practices. Works with energy balancing.

Primary Muscle—The muscle that is in use in that movement.

Prone—Lying on your stomach/chest.

Protraction—Straightforward.

Proximal—Situated toward the point of attachment.

Psychiatrist—A doctor who does prescribe medicine for issues in the brain and thought/behavior patterns.

Psychologist—A therapist who does not prescribe medication but does help you get to the root cause of things. There is no hands-on in this practice. It is talk therapy based. Trained in counseling.

Qi Gong—"Life energy cultivation" through slow movements, postures, breathing, and more. Qi Gong (pronounced chi gong) is used to cultivate chi or life force energy.

Reflexology—Originated with the Chinese zone theory. It works with the feet to access and affect organs throughout the body.

Reiki—Developed in Japan and used in hospitals in Japan to this day. This is much like therapeutic touch. It is a laying of the hands to balance and realign the energy channels of the body. I use this practice to help people get to an emotional release. The energy can help you release things that do not serve your highest good, and replenish the areas with unconditional love. The facilitator is simply a channel from spirit to you.

Retraction—Straight backward.

Rolfing—Developed by Ida Rolf. This is a method to realign the body in relationship to gravity. It frees up fascia and chronic tension patterns. It is considered a bit rough in its delivery, but highly effective. If your body has issues with chronic misalignments, this is ideal.

Secondary muscle—The muscle that has to turn off in order for the opposing muscle to turn on.

Shaman—Native American medicine person. Can use many techniques for healing. Herbs, soul retrieval, extraction, prayer, and ritual. Can heal many root issues and help you to serve the earth as your best self.

Shiatsu—A modern Japanese system based on the meridians and Asian philosophy. It involves pressure on acupoints and various other physical manipulations to affect the flow of energy.

Superior—Upper body.

Supine—Lying on your back.

Tai Chi—"Supreme ultimate boxing" is a martial art originating in China. It is a combination of self-defense as well as slow movements to help bring mental clarity and calm. Tai chi helps the body heal down to the marrow of the bone. It is extremely beneficial in healing and can be applied to any population.

Thai Massage—Assisted stretching. This is done on a mat on the ground. For the client, it is passive. The facilitator does all the work and you feel all the results!

Thai Yoga Therapy—A system that incorporates Thai massage with yoga practice. It involves yoga postures, twisting, and stretching led by a therapist.

Therapeutic Touch—"Non-contact therapeutic touch" is the formal definition. A person uses his or her hands to affect the energy field around someone but not with direct skin to skin touch.

Tao—(pronounced dow) Is a Chinese term that loosely means "the way." It is a spiritual practice.

Watsu—Is a massage/stretching technique done while lying in warm water. The treatment is continuously supported by the therapist as they rock and gently stretch the body. The body is free to be manipulated and stretched in ways impossible while on land.

Yoga—Translates to union of your three selves—the physical self, the conscious self, and the higher self. It is a combination of physical postures, breathing, chanting, meditation, and diet.

Bibliography

Crosswell, AD, Bower JE, Ganz PA. "Childhood Adversity and Inflammation in Breast Cancer Survivors." *Psychosomatic medicine* 76(3), (April 2014): 208–214. doi:10.1097/PSY.0000000000000041.

Dharmananda, Subhuti. "How Emotions May Contribute to Cancer." September 1999. http://www.itmonline.org/arts/cancemo.htm.

"Evolution of Consciousness." Evolution of Consciousness. http://www.consciousawareness.info/meridians.

Fuller-Thomson, Esme, and Sarah Brennenstuhl. "Making a Link between Childhood Physical Abuse and Cancer." *Cancer* 115, no. 14 (2009): 3341–350. doi:10.1002/cncr.24372.

Goldsmith RE, Jandorf L, Valdimarsdottir H, et al. "Traumatic stress symptoms and breast cancer: The role of childhood abuse." *Child Abuse & Neglect* 34(6) (2010):465–470. doi:10.1016/j.chiabu.2009.10.007.

Hạnh, Nhất, and Robert Ellsberg. *Thich Nhat Hanh: Essential Writings*. Maryknoll, NY: Orbis Books, 2001.

Keleman, Stanley. *Emotional Anatomy: The Structure of Experience*. Berkeley, CA: Center Press, 1985.

———. *Your Body Speaks Its Mind: The Bio-energetic Way to Greater Emotional and Sexual Satisfaction*. New York: Simon and Schuster, 1975.

Kaptchuk, Ted J. *The Web That Has No Weaver: Understanding Chinese Medicine*. New York: Congdon & Weed, 1983.

Natural Health Zone. "The Body Meridians." Natural Health Zone. http://www.natural-health-zone.com/body-meridians.html.

National Cancer Institute. "Psychological Stress and Cancer." National Cancer Institute. December 10, 2012. https://www.cancer.gov/about-cancer/coping/feelings/stress-fact-sheet.

Schnur, J. B., and R. E. Goldsmith. "Through Her Eyes." *Journal of Clinical Oncology* 29, no. 30 (2011): 4054–056. doi:10.1200/jco.2011.37.2409.

Stringer, Heather. "Unlocking the Emotions of Cancer." *PsycEXTRA Dataset.* doi:10.1037/e573082014-011.

Wilbanks, Brett. "The 'Muscle of the Soul' May Be Triggering Your Fear and Anxiety." The Mind Unleashed. July 6, 2015. http://themindunleashed.com/2015/07/the-muscle-of-the-soul-may-be-triggering-your-fear-and-anxiety.html.

Wise, LA, JR Palmer, DA Boggs, LL Adams-Campbell, and L Rosenberg. "Abuse victimization and risk of breast cancer in the Black Women's Health Study: Abuse and breast cancer risk in black women." 22(4), (2011): 659–669. doi:10.1007/s10552-011-9738-3.

Witek Janusek, L, D Tell, K Albuquerque, HL Mathews. "Childhood adversity increases vulnerability for behavioral symptoms and immune dysregulation in women with breast cancer." *Brain, behavior, and immunity* 30(Suppl), (2013): S149–S162. doi:10.1016/j.bbi.2012.05.014.

Wolfe, David. "Study: Burning Sage (Smudging) Can Eliminate Harmful Air Pollutants." David Wolfe. https://www.davidwolfe.com/burning-sage-smudging/?c=pwf&vp=dchop.

Index

To Write to the Author

If you wish to contact the author or would like more information about this book, please write to the author in care of Llewellyn Worldwide Ltd. and we will forward your request. Both the author and publisher appreciate hearing from you and learning of your enjoyment of this book and how it has helped you. Llewellyn Worldwide Ltd. cannot guarantee that every letter written to the author can be answered, but all will be forwarded. Please write to:

Emily A. Francis
℅ Llewellyn Worldwide
2143 Wooddale Drive
Woodbury, MN 55125-2989

Please enclose a self-addressed stamped envelope for reply,
or $1.00 to cover costs. If outside the U.S.A., enclose
an international postal reply coupon.

Many of Llewellyn's authors have websites with additional information and resources. For more information, please visit our website at http://www.llewellyn.com